Medicine For The Coming Age

Dr Lisa Sand

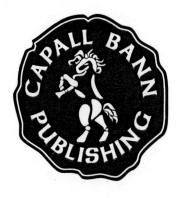

Medicine For The Coming Age

Author: Lisa Sand MD
in collaboration with
Mary Russell BSc BA (Hons) Psychology

ISBN 186163 068 9

Cover design by Paul Mason

Published by:

Capall Bann Publishing
Freshfields
Chieveley
Berks
RG20 8TF

Dedication

to the spirit of man on earth for whom this manuscript is intended by the great souls who have taught me from the level of Reality and who refer to it as "our book".

Inga Hooper is now one of them.

Acknowledgements

Many heartfelt thanks to Mary Russell

for her great help and support;

and to

Suzy Reid

for her indefatigable patience in preparing and expediting
material for the publishers

and to Jo Barber

for finding the right publisher

Contents

Foreword

This book covers some of the clinical experience collected by Dr. Sand in her collaboration with a fine medium and a number of experts in the 'world unseen'.

The experiment extended over a period of twenty-three years in two countries. Basic to it has been the awareness that man is not his body and his personality but an external part of the Creator. Without this recognition he is in trouble with himself and his surroundings, but if he can make peace between his personality and his true being he will 'live happily ever after'.

This state of harmony escapes him as long as he is plagued by old thoughts buried, however deeply, in his consciousness and resulting from traumatic experiences and indoctrinations which he has taken on board. They must be brought out and seen in the light of day in order to be dispersed. A feeling of liberation from bondage is the result together with abundant humour and laughter. Dr. Sand and her visible and invisible team have usually achieved such a result in record time.

Dr. Sand's book is also an inspired document. Like her work it is the result of collaboration with discarnate experts. The book is a handbook of human psychology, the study of the soul, as it is. There is no dogma or pet human misconceptions, only a statement of the facts as seen from the dimension of reality and put into practice by Dr. Sand and her team.

Mary Russell Bsc, BA (Hons) Psychology

"Man know thyself"

Grateful acknowledgement is given
to the inspiration of
Prof. Carl Gustav Jung

Section 1

Soul Directed Therapy

Chapter 1

A Definition of Spiritual Psychotherapy

Spiritual psychotherapy fully recognises the three-fold nature of man, body, mind and soul. It is aware that the soul of man is not limited by time and space, that it is "in the world but not of it". As an entity of a higher dimension of being it seeks the unfoldment of experience through expression in the temporary restriction we call body, with its mind and psyche.

Reincarnation is also accepted as a fact and with it the knowledge that the soul has had many different embodiments as both men and women in the course of the centuries. Accompanying this realisation is the awareness of the immutable law of cause and effect which governs the entire universe and in it the lives of human beings.

Spiritual psychotherapy recognises pain and suffering as stimuli, driving the afflicted person into activity towards inner progress. It is said that nature abhors a vacuum. Similarly, it may be said that the soul abhors stagnation. When a painful stimulus has served its purpose for the soul of the sufferer or for those in his environment for whom it was intended, it becomes a hindrance to further progression if it is not resolved or removed, as it then hampers the free expression of the soul through body and psyche, often referred to as the "vehicle". A person so afflicted may seek help to improve the condition and may be brought into contact with the spiritual psychotherapist.

Being aware of the soul or spirit as eternal, the therapist is also cognisant of the existence of beings who are not at the moment attached to an earthly body. Among them are experienced psychotherapists who, from the far greater wisdom and breadth of a consciousness unobstructed by matter, are eager to assist the spiritual psychotherapist in his work by their thought directed into his own thinking and that of his patients.

Spiritual psychotherapy is not bound by the limitations of any particular school or method of psychotherapy. It can freely make use of the content of any or all of them depending upon the particular needs of the patient and the special abilities of the therapist. It is also free to use any method or approach hitherto regarded as lying outside the province of psychotherapy as long as the action is wisely conceived to produce the desired therapeutic result.

Not being limited by any system, the new treatment may suddenly switch from one approach to another, should it become evident that the element of surprise or the startled reaction of the patient will facilitate his letting go of a particular emotional attitude like stubbornness, rebellion or self-pity.

I am not creating a new school or system of psychotherapy with a founder or originator who gathers about himself devotees to his method who hang on all his pronouncements and seek to emulate them for ever after. No, the new therapy could be called open-ended. Every talented person active in the field works according to his or her own light and meets with colleagues for a free give-and-take of original contributions and experience. The only valid criterion is the success of treatment and the safety of the patient under the therapist's care.

These conditions are designed to assure rapid growth of therapeutic knowledge through a free flow of information between workers in the field, permitting the development of revolutionary procedures in the hands of those equipped to carry them out successfully. A free and easy give-and-take also tends to avoid fossilisation and stagnation. The open-ended method rides upon the crest of the wave, moving freely with changing requirements.

Chapter 2

Requirements for being a Spiritual Psychotherapist

The prospective candidate for becoming a spiritual psychotherapist must, regardless of age, have suffered enough in his life to have developed considerable humility and the ability to understand the suffering and difficulties of others with compassion. Preparation for doing the work must have taken place in previous existences on earth, so that there is a much vaster range of experience to draw upon than anyone can ever gather in one lifetime. The candidate need not actually remember those prior incarnations. He will, however, feel a sense of mission within himself. Often he will have noticed, even from childhood, that people turned to him with various problems under a wide variety of circumstances. He will have felt a deep sense of gratitude and joy whenever he has been able to help someone who has turned to him in this way. A strong desire to help many more will on occasion enter the consciousness of such a one, at times already at a surprisingly young age, at other times not until middle age has brought great upheavals in the life pattern.

Along with humility and compassion there must be a basic honesty in the character of the candidate. On the basis of this honesty, he must realise that he has had problems himself and has had the courage to seek help toward the resolution of these problems in a straight-forward fashion. In this connection it is noteworthy that a relatively large number of candidates have made not one but a number of active attempts to find someone or some system to help them rid themselves of their emotional difficulties and repetitive neurotic behaviour problems. Usually success has been at best partial until they have found their way to a spiritual psychotherapist. Some have become conscious of their own calling only through the liberation from their disorder during individual treatment.

Once the would-be therapist has been freed from his own conditioning and the deep-seated anxieties due to it he must be able and willing to treat others with loving compassion but without any emotional involvement. This requires a degree of maturity found only in a relatively old soul which may, however, reside in a young body.

Of great importance in the character of the spiritual psychotherapist is a sense of responsibility. There should be considerable evidence of this quality in his life up to the present time. This sense of responsibility is not to be confused with a neurotic kind of guilt-ridden and compulsive adherence to a concept of duty.

Most candidates are aware of invisible, hereafter referred to as "higher dimensional", influences, connections, guidance etc., even before they receive their own treatment. Others discover their spiritual sensitivity somewhat later. All must be honest enough to have an open mind, regardless of popular prejudice and opinion. They must learn to be true to their innermost selves; have the courage of their convictions, and take a stand with others of a like mind.

If the above criteria of character and intentions are fulfilled, the candidate should then acquire a basic knowledge of psychological mechanisms and diagnostic criteria. This can be done quite rapidly by a talented individual. Some have such information already or wish to go into more formal training of a professional nature in order to qualify for regular employment. Some are professionally active in other fields of endeavour, using their therapeutic ability part-time or as the occasion arises. There are no restrictive rules and regulations imposed on spiritual psychotherapists by their own colleagues. They are simply expected to remain true to their responsibility, to the inner self and to their patients.

An educational level affording a good to excellent general vocabulary and the ability to concentrate are most desirable attributes. A fine intelligence is necessary; but here it must be said that some have been conditioned to regard themselves as unintelligent and discover their actual level only in the course of their own treatment. This requisite intelligence is not to be confused with intellectuality or book learning. It is, rather, an innate inner wisdom.

The humility necessary in the character of the spiritual psychotherapist rests upon the knowledge that he is, and functions simply as, the instrument of a higher power and came into this life prepared to serve. There must be the willingness and the desire to subjugate his lower or outer self to his higher self and to trust its infinitely greater wisdom, love and experience.

In order to understand himself in a proper perspective, it is often necessary that the future therapist not only rids himself of faulty conditioning received in his early life but also that he recollects or has brought to his attention salient features of one or more embodiments preceding his present one. This gives him a considerably more broadened view of the law of cause and effect. It helps him to understand himself much better and to be less short-sighted in regard to others.

A sense of humour and of fun will greatly enhance the work process. It serves to restore perspective at critical moments, having a heart-warming and relaxing effect. Spiritual man is neither solemn nor "holy". He is always ready for laughter and is fun-loving.

A high degree of flexibility is also a necessary character trait of the spiritual psychotherapist. He is constantly confronted by changing, often surprising turns of thoughts, feelings, and events in connection with his patients and, of course, also in his own life. He must be able to rise to these occasions, demonstrating a level of maturity which will serve as a living example to all who have contact with him.

A spiritually aware person welcomes change as the necessary pre-condition for progress, and as positive proof that no stagnation has set in. He knows that learning and becoming depend upon the active handling of the changing situations and conditions as they present themselves. His basic knowledge of cosmic law regarding thought and action should make flexibility easy rather than difficult and cause him to realise that his own continued inner growth and development is an absolute necessity to avoid stagnation which can only result in the devaluation of his role as a therapist.

If the reader feels that the requirements mentioned in this chapter relating to the character and life experience of the spiritual psychotherapist are too stringent, then let him meditate on what he himself, as a patient, would like to see in one whom he would honestly bare his innermost thoughts. How would he feel about putting his trust in one who could say: "Do as I say; don't do as I do!" ?

Chapter 3

Who are the Patients Coming to the Spiritual Psychotherapist?

The people requesting help cannot possibly be classed as belonging to one or another type. They will represent every conceivable kind of background, culture, race, nation, education, and age. As long as the therapist is in good connection with his own inner source of inspiration the range of patients most likely to profit from his particular skill will find their way to him and he will enjoy working with them. He will marvel at the often amazing ways in which patients are directed to him. At times, he will have the feeling that his life is a series of fairy tales.

The problems and difficulties with which patients arrive will be myriad. These difficulties will express themselves in the emotional and thinking processes, in interpersonal relationships, life situations, attitudes, physical symptoms, and even the consequences of misuse of psychic and mediumistic abilities. The patient may or may not be aware of being more than a body with a brain. He has to be dealt with on his own level of understanding which is often not that of the therapist. A patient who is burdened beyond his readiness to grasp spiritual information will be confused, bewildered, and even angered. Such a situation will add to his load of anxiety rather than reduce it. In any case, the therapist must see himself as a channel and leave the selection of patients guided to him to the same higher source from which he receives his own inspiration.

With increasing experience, the devoted and talented therapist will undoubtedly be employed more and more to treat others who, like himself, have come into this life to serve in a similar fashion. The number of such souls ready for "clearance" is rapidly increasing.

The future therapist should realise that, to be most effective, he should be more than willing to work in a team with others who share a similar sense of purpose. Where the devotion to service is steady and strong, Centres are likely to be established to simplify treatment from which will grow teaching and other related activities. This type of arrangement is already foreseen by the higher dimensional level on an international scale for the New Age.

Chapter 4

The Goals of Treatment

The goal to be achieved with the individual patient and the therapist working together must be thoroughly flexible. It depends only partly on the therapist and to a large extent on the patient. Some general statements, however, may be made. It is a fact that the more love and optimism shines out of the therapist, the more the patient feels motivated to achieve the most of which he is capable in the betterment of his condition. The patient's own higher Self will take maximum advantage of the opportunity offered to get its vehicle into harmonious working order, so that the patient will feel a great drive within himself to progress rapidly and extensively in the presence of a truly positive therapist.

When the latter is in good touch with his own source he will not make mistakes regarding goals. He will even be able to influence the patient's own goal if it is too modest. The "tuned-in" therapist will have no difficulty in assessing the situation from moment to moment, as he need not rely on his own personal intellect exclusively but lets himself be carried along by the much greater intelligence and vision of the skilled souls working through the instrument of his consciousness.

At times, there will be a long pause between treatment sessions in a particular case as it becomes necessary for the patient to accumulate life experience with his own newly extended vision before he is ready for further change through treatment. Here again the therapist is expected to have total flexibility and simply submit to the management by a higher level of consciousness, even if he does not understand the reasons at the time. When the patient is ready to resume treatment, the therapist will accept him again with the same positivity as before.

Patients will be of different degrees of maturity of soul. The possible level of achievement will vary accordingly. Health and wholeness for one person will consist of a simple, cheerful getting along in the home and job situation; for another person it will mean the active use of an innate artistic ability or service to many others in healing or administration of some sort according to some special talent of which he might previously have been unaware. Quite often a patient will make major changes in his life situation, in the personal and professional spheres, on the basis of insights gained in the course of his treatment. Let it be said that the responsibility of the therapist to his patient rests in helping him to the insights he needs to make his own decisions on a sound and rational basis, NOT to make them for him. He should recognise when the patient is ready and able to decide from a mature basis. Until such time the therapist may have to ask the patient to postpone deciding till later.

At times a goal envisaged at the beginning of treatment turns out to have been quite unrealistic in one or the other direction. Using his own free will, the patient may make an amazing jump forward or go into a rebellious stance which he will not relinquish. The latter can usually be bridged over if the therapist is very positive and has a good sense of humour which can stimulate the patient's own sense of the ridiculous.

Unexpected turns in the therapeutic approach to the patient or in the patient's response to treatment can instantaneously cause the goal to change. Great flexibility makes the course of treatment interesting, even fascinating, and certainly eliminates periods of stagnation.

On a deeper level the goal of treatment in the end is the clearing away of all blockages in the psyche to a perfectly free flow of energies. Expressed differently, one can call it a centering of the individual or a harmonisation of all his constituent abilities in a multi-dimensional whole. It is a synchronisation of the lower self with the higher Self so that they form a unit, a one-ness, with the spirit in command at all times and in all things big and small, inner and outer. This is what natural man represented until the ravages of man-made civilisation, with all its negative conditioning, exploded his at-one-ment with himself, with all of nature, and all of spirit. He knew himself to be part of the Whole, not apart from it.

Chapter 5

Treatment

The "how" of treatment is guided by quite simple general principles. When the conditions mentioned in previous chapters are fulfilled patients come to the therapist in various degrees of anxious expectation. Some have high hopes because they have seen the benefit someone else has received; some are hopeful but bracing themselves against yet another failure in their search for relief. Others hide their hurt, sensitivity, and vulnerability behind one or another facade. Some talk like a waterfall, others hardly get a word out. There are as many variants as there are people.

The therapist must radiate calm, cheerful composure, confidence, and a deep caring. In this way he has an immediate tranquilising effect on the patient's initial anxiety. If the patient is under pressure of speech, the therapist will just listen in an interested way until there is a pause and a question is warranted. A psychotherapist must be a good listener at all times, with plenty of patience.

If the patient has difficulty speaking, the therapist must ask him about his reasons for coming and encourage him to talk. Routine questioning should not be overdone as much information can be gleaned later. Depending on the particular situation, routine questioning may be virtually abandoned during the first visit according to the motto "First things first". Here, too, flexibility is desirable.

I consider it of the foremost importance that the patient should have some beneficial result from every meeting with the therapist, especially the first one. Even if this effect should at first be only short-lived, the patient should leave the therapist's presence with a feeling of upliftment, a realisation that he understands himself better than he did when he came in, and an awareness that he has been understood.

About two hours should be allotted for such a first session, one and a half hours being an absolute minimum. It may be impossible to achieve a therapeutic effect in less time and this effect is necessary to allay some of the patient's apprehensions about the treatment situation. It also makes him feel that there is hope for him and that his difficulties are neither as unique nor as mysterious as they have seemed to him. He feels better about himself and thus sees himself in a more favourable light than before.

During the first interview the patient is generally informed that in treatment he will come to know himself; that it is not important how much the therapist finds out about him, but that the patient begins to understand his own attitudes, actions, symptoms, feelings, thoughts and expectations, so that he can become the "captain of his ship" in fuller awareness, rather than be blown back and forth by unknown forces.

Very rarely there may be a patient whose problem is sufficiently superficial to be actually cleared up on the very first visit. This situation would pertain to a basically mature individual who has not overcome some traumatic event in his adult life because he has not been honest with himself about something or someone in regard to this occurrence.

The second interview should generally be arranged as close as possible in time to the first one, so that there will be no real loss of momentum between the two. All through the course of treatment there should be flexibility regarding the frequency of sessions. Given the practical feasibility, it may at times be of advantage to meet daily, while at other times an interval of a week may be desirable, so that the patient can test out his newly acquired insights and self-confidence in daily life before going on further. Gains are consolidated in this fashion toward the end of treatment.

In spiritual psychotherapy well done, progress is at times so rapid that the patient needs some time to get used to his new self, a process amusing to behold and to experience. It involves not only feelings and attitudes on the part of the patient but also their startling effect on the persons in his environment, their responsiveness to him.

Most of the therapist's time during treatment is spent in attentive and relaxed listening. This alternates with questions asked of the patient designed to help him discover the roots and ramifications of his attitudes and behaviour. By letting the patient digress as his associations happen to lead him, valuable connections and patterns are brought to light, to his astonishment. Sooner or later patients will see the origin of their repetitive and distorted behaviour, experiences and emotions in the real or phantasized circumstances and relationships of their early and later childhood. During the process of bringing these to the surface of consciousness it becomes evident that the memory of some events had been repressed out of awareness at an early stage. Sometimes the memory remained but its emotional content had become unconscious, influencing from its hidden recess the patient's thoughts, actions, and decisions to a remarkable extent, often causing calamities and heartache and keeping him from unfolding his real potential in life.

Mary, a twenty-four year old entertainer, illustrated these mechanisms very well. She had married at nineteen, was divorced at twenty-two. At twenty-three she made several suicide attempts, some almost successfully. At the end of one year these attempts stopped as suddenly as they had begun. A year of conventional psychotherapy had not resulted in any noticeable change. Soon after the suicide attempts ceased, Mary developed acute rheumatoid arthritis, a badly crippling disease. She spent four months in a hospital, receiving the usual treatment with corticoids. Soon after her release she came to see me. She was working again but the arthritis continued to be active at intervals. There was already a mild degree of visible deformity in some joints, a very serious problem for a professional entertainer. Mary came to see me twice, each time about two hours, and the following history emerged: When she was ten years old, her brother, on his twenty-first birthday, drove the father's tractor recklessly, turning it over onto himself. He was instantly killed. Mary was nearby but did not see the accident itself.

In Mary's childhood home there was very little positive communication between the members of the family, but an overconcern with material matters and considerable harshness. The young man had been the only son. Mary knew that she had had an argument with her brother the evening preceding the fatal accident. In lending emphasis to her statements she had said to him: "And I hope you die", as she had said on previous occasions also, though she was quite fond of him.

As she spoke with me, it was obvious that she had never forgotten these events. However, in her second session with me she realised to her amazement and shock that, following her brother's death, she had in her phantasy, taken herself to task and decided that through her words of ". . . and I hope you die", she had magically become his murderess, as those words had obviously been a command to destiny. The child, raised in an environment of impoverished communications, spoke to no-one about her terrible secret and the deep feelings of guilt and sorrow it engendered. Since the thought and the emotions were both intolerable, they were promptly "forgotten", that means repressed into the unconscious. Mary had forthwith lost all awareness of them. Only the memory of the accident and the quarrels remained.

Fourteen years later the emergence of the submerged guilt phantasy brought into focus the why and wherefore of the apparently disconnected events of her life in these years. In her teens she had become surprisingly interested in agricultural science, taking courses as early as possible, in order to be of help to her father on the farm. She now realised that she wanted to atone to him for the "murder" of his only son. At nineteen she married a farmer whose land adjoined her father's, so that her husband could work on both properties. In my presence she realised for the first time that this marriage was another unconscious attempt at restitution to her father.

Needless to say, this marriage was bound to fail as there was no real basis on which it could thrive. The couple separated, divorced. As Mary approached her twenty-first birthday, she told friends she felt certain that she would not live beyond that date, though she couldn't tell why. But the day came and went quite uneventfully. Now three years later, Mary could see that on the basis of unconscious magic thinking she was certain that "fate" would execute a death sentence on her for the murder of her brother.

At no time did Mary regret her divorce. Professionally she was quite satisfied. She could see no particular reason for her suicide attempts, stating that she could not say that they were the result of depression. Her words to me were: "I just felt like it". After her recollection of the repressed phantasy she easily recognised that the suicide attempts were again a matter of trying to carry out the death penalty to which she had sentenced herself. After a year of failures to succeed, they stopped.

I was then able to help Mary to comprehend that the crippling arthritis constituted yet another severe sentence she had meted out to herself and would henceforth disappear as adult reason did away with the uncovered cause.

Mary has never been back to see me since that day. She changed jobs just then and her new work schedule did not make further visits possible. For some weeks she telephoned regularly to report on her progress. She said she felt as if a big, heavy stone had been removed from her back. It took her several weeks to become used to its absence because it had been there so long. Having had a continuous feeling of tenseness all those years, she now enjoyed laughing as she hadn't done all that time. She made some changes in her life situation in the following months.

When a patient resents having been born into untoward, harsh circumstances or having had painful experiences early in life, he sees himself as the innocent victim of a distorted adult world. The therapist then has to explain a bit about the great law of cause and effect , as far as the patient's understanding allows it, pointing out that only the body was young. The soul had been gathering experience for aeons. Quite often it is possible to recognise what lessons it has to learn in the present life. Where there is no actual memory of other incarnations, the mere knowledge that the circumstances of the present one are a direct consequence of the soul's handling of those in other lifetimes is often very helpful.

When deeply submerged emotional material is brought to light by the patient, there is often a rather violent outburst with weeping and sobbing, at times followed by laughter. The inexperienced therapist may be frightened by such a scene if he did not have any during his own treatment. These reactions constitute a great release and are followed by a sensation of liberation on the spot.

As the therapist's attention is focussed on the patient, his utterings and his emotional tone must be taken notice of, particularly any feelings of lack of self-esteem, guilt feelings, and also any train of thought which can only pull the patient down without serving a constructive purpose. The self-image must be cleverly supported and built-up by the therapist, and damaging and destructive tendencies modified into positive forces for constructive action.

Resistances to the unearthing of repressed emotional material are amply described in psycho-analytic literature. They are a normal part of deep insight therapy, as there is always a portion of the psyche which is dreadfully afraid of the unknown submerged emotions. The resistances take many forms. It is to be noted that material was originally suppressed because it was so painful and overwhelming at the time that it threatened the very integrity of the personality. Obviously, then, the repression constituted a valuable defence mechanism in the face of intolerable odds. Resistance stems from this original, usually childish terror. It is not to be despised, but understood. The therapist's inspirers will know how to deal with even the most tenacious cases in quite a variety of ways.

There are other defensive mechanisms such as conversion, which is the transforming of anxiety into a physical symptom. In projection, inner disharmonies and conflicts are seen as occurring in or through other people. Introjection sees traits and attitudes of someone important in the immediate environment as being part of self. At their inception, all those defence mechanisms were applied in an attempt to hold the personality together. Thus they constitute outworn props, usually from early childhood, which have to be replaced by a wholesome self-esteem as they are removed.

Another mechanism, well-known in psycho-analysis, is so-called negative transference. This is peculiar to the treatment situation. The patient unconsciously sees the therapist as one or another of the important adults in his childhood and reacts and behaves accordingly. The therapist must not respond to the patient's negative attitudes on an emotional basis. They can be used to increase the patient's awareness very substantially. By the same token the therapist must be immune to flattery used as a resistance in the sense of: "If I flatter you, you'll spare me the hurt of taking a look at my unconscious content".

The therapist must be familiar with the use of symbols. Dream analysis furnishes a short-cut to the unconscious, and the patient must be helped to de-symbolise or uncode his dreams. Even if, at times, the therapist immediately knows the meaning of a dream, it is usually advisable that the patient works it out for himself, with the necessary help, as the effect is much stronger this way. It is also to be remembered that one and the same symbol can mean different things to different people and even at different times to the same person.

In contrast to the traditional psycho-analyst, the spiritual psychotherapist is aware that dreams are of different kinds and have diverse origins. There are even experiences which are not dreams at all but out-of-body journeys from which a more or less distorted memory is brought back into the physical consciousness. Most dreams are of the common or garden variety which deals with wish-fulfilments, unresolved conflicts, problem situations, and anxieties. They serve a purpose by supplying easy access to hidden problem areas in the psyche, circumventing some resistances on the road to greater insight. However, there are some dreams, usually short, which are obviously planted by the person's own higher consciousness. They are usually easy of interpretation and frequently show a remarkable sense of humour in the deciphered content and the choice of symbols. Into this category fits the dream of a patient with ample black hair who, one night, had an encounter with a beautiful black panther who obviously loved him very much. The animal nipped him in the hand once. The patient told it not to do that any more and go out of the house and not come back; but the panther kept returning through special openings in the doors, behaving most lovingly. Upon analysis it was clear that the patient saw his own higher Self as the beautiful big cat. Because of a misconception, namely that letting it govern his actions and attitudes meant being "holy", he was resisting its take-over, didn't trust it. Interpreting the dream led to the immediate removal of the misconception and merry laughter.

Occasionally, patients have had prophetic dreams during their lives. These most often announce rather unimportant events and situations, being startling only by their accuracy of detail. Rarely, they have to do with important things, mostly painful ones. The spiritual therapist knows that neither time nor space are what they appear to be to mortal man and, therefore, accepts the existence of "advance" knowledge without difficulty. These relatively unusual dream experiences are very clear and are not quickly and easily forgotten as are most ordinary dreams.

Yet another variety of non-dream is the recollection of scenes or sequences from other life-times or even of the process of incarnation itself. These are also remembered with great clarity for indefinite periods of time. In the main, however, the therapist will deal with the common, the "real" dream. He will have learned that colours in dreams have to do with the emotional and feeling content and that thoughts and emotions following the dream or upon awakening are to be treated as part of it. Everything and every person, as well as any detail contained in a dream is highly symbolic. The dream does not represent what it appears to state. "Confused" dreams are just as analysable as those which appear to tell a coherent story. The therapist helps the patient to do his own deciphering of the dream. The hidden content must ring true to the dreamer himself, otherwise it is without value. While working out a dream, the patient may go far afield in his self-discovery, often arriving at the actual dream content by a circuitous route. The process must be experienced in order to be understood.

Alice dreamt of a partly dismantled car several times. She described the vehicle as grey, cold, metallic and in unfriendly surroundings. Upon deciphering the dream, the car turned out to represent both her father and her lover. Both had been unable to show her any real love and affection. She had even consciously realised similarities between the two men. The father had died before she was grown up. The dream expressed her realisation that the lover, like the father, would not change, that she had simply repeated the childhood experience, as so frequently happens before the patient has received treatment. The fact that the car was partially dismantled showed her feeling that both men were, in a way, incomplete. They could not even love properly in the state they were in. The unfriendly surroundings, which were represented differently each time the dream recurred, indicated the fact that each of the two men had brought unhappiness not only to her but also to others associated with them. The patient realised the necessity of breaking away from her lover. Soon her condition had improved to the point where she was no longer in danger of repeating the childhood experience with other men.

Not only the patient's dreams, but all his symptoms and his symptomatic behaviour are symbolic in one way or another. It is the therapist's task to enable the patient to recognise these patterns in their true meaning. Discovering their roots in the patient's past experience is absolutely necessary for their relief.

Michael had for many years been suffering from frequent colds, sore throats and 'flu's. In the course of his treatment he came to realise that, as a child, he had not received the love and affection which a little one needs to develop normally. However, when he happened to be ill his mother became concerned and hovered over him. This extra attention was the nearest thing to affectionate love he could obtain. Quite logically, he came down with infections quite frequently thereafter. Now, as an adult, the recognition of the old pattern and the insight that his needs could be fulfilled in quite another way freed him from further repetitions of the illnesses. Patients are often surprised and appaled to find out how much of their behaviour and thinking derives from the conditioning they have received, especially in their childhood and youth. This is easy to understand, however, if one realises that the effectiveness of advertising and propaganda of any sort is dependent upon man's suggestibility. Once the patient has fully understood the problem areas of conditioning in himself he can eliminate them and can safeguard himself against future such assaults by his own intelligence and self assertion.

A powerful form of conditioning is the planting of suggestions, which can be done in quite a subtle fashion. In this respect it behoves the psychotherapist to be aware of his great responsibility. He must not plant ideas which could possibly have negative effects. This is a major reason why he should be "sorted-out" before he works with patients in depth. Otherwise, he is not a clear channel for his inspirers and will impress some of his own conditioned thinking on the patient, causing confusion or even panic instead of creating clarity and peace.

When dealing with patients who are acquainted with the value of mediumship I often avail myself of the services of an experienced, reliable clairaudient and clairvoyant. This highly trained and prepared sensitive has herself been "cleared" and is, therefore, eminently suitable to assist in such work. The patients who have benefited from this unusual collaboration have been very grateful for it indeed. The sensitive, hereafter referred to as the "mediator", the patient and I, on these occasions sit together in the treatment room without any formality. The mediator is used to transmit most valuable information and counsel from "dead" relatives or advisers of the patient and the fourth dimension. Even if the patient is not immediately able to make full use of the material thus received, I make notes of it and use it subsequently in the treatment. This extraordinary procedure cuts many corners, streamlining the course of therapy. Many times, in these special sessions with the mediator, I have seen strong resistance or rebellion in the patient vanish after a major emotional release.

Since consciousness has many dimensions, the spiritual psychotherapist can have no misgivings about a free and easy give-and-take between the dimensions whenever there is the opportunity and the need. He knows that basically all is one, and will not close his mind to the myriad possibilities and variations of treatment available under different circumstances. He will reap a rich harvest of joyous satisfaction and fulfilment through keeping an open mind. The awareness of his own higher receptive senses will also be furthered by this attitude, as he becomes a more and more valuable instrument for those in the higher dimensions who are ready to work through and with him to transmute the negativity existing in human thinking and feeling.

The therapist must ever keep in mind that the patient's spirit has learned from all life-experience. No experience is to be despised, therefore. In most instances the patient is made aware of the specific value of what has happened to him. A major purpose of treatment is to enable the patient to relinquish his negative emotional attachment to events and people of his past and present, whether this emotional involvement has been conscious or unconscious. Upon such release he is then able to learn the lesson inherent in the experiences and, thus, put a stop to their repetition in one or another form. These repetitions often remind the observer of a cracked phonograph record playing the same groove over and over again. Like the phonograph needle which has been lifted over the defect, the freed individual is finally able to go on to new and different life experiences and opportunities for progression.

When a patient resents the fact that he was exposed to great harshness and apparent injustice in childhood, leading to trouble in his unfoldment and in his search for identity, the therapist may have to point out to him the inexorable working out of the great law of cause and effect. The patient must learn to understand and accept that his life did not begin at birth; that merely the body was new, not the soul. If he has no actual memory of having lived before such recollection or information may be given to him so that he may perceive that the circumstances of the present life are a direct and logical consequence of the soul's handling of the circumstances in other lifetimes through the vehicle it then occupied.

Nothing and nobody on earth is free of error. Thus, the spiritual psychotherapist is not always perfectly attuned to his source and makes occasional mistakes like everyone else. That is not important if he is at all times willing to admit and correct his error as soon as he becomes aware of it or his attention is drawn to it. A sense of humour and proportion is helpful in this as in every other respect.

No therapist must ever forget his absolute duty to guard the confidentiality of what he has heard or found out regarding his patients and of their identity. Secrecy of this kind is standard in the medical, legal and allied professions. A breach of confidence can never be repaired and is a source of painful embarrassment.

The importance of dignity must always be remembered. Spiritual man has a natural dignity at all times and will automatically support and enhance the selfhood of all with whom he comes in contact. The spiritual psychotherapist should observe the difference between real natural dignity and affectedness of one or another sort. The latter generally hides a more or less deep feeling of inadequacy, a fear, or an attempt to show off.

Positive thinking is a great power. The therapist must use it with his patients. Even if he feels a bit dismayed at times, he must not take this feeling seriously, nor focus his attention on it. It will then pass in a moment. With increasing experience he will find out that hardly a soul is not helped by his efforts as long as he remains "in touch" and positive in attitude and conviction in his own being. At times he may feel that he has not been able to do much for someone he has seen only once or twice, only to hear later that the person concerned has revolutionised his attitudes and circumstances of living. Every insight is helpful toward progress. By the time a patient has found his way to the therapist he is ready to take a good look at himself. This means that the therapist's optimistic outlook rests on a very firm foundation when he works with those who have voluntarily come to him. This real confidence is also sensed and incorporated by the patient and used on his own behalf. No bravado is necessary or desirable. A quiet assuredness and verbal reassurance if indicated is all that is required.

Ever since civilised man has established a custom of making laughter incumbent upon the telling of jokes or witticisms he has forgotten that for natural man laughing is an expression of joy and pleasure not in any way dependent on something being funny, witty or ridiculous. Here again a natural function designed to keep body and soul functioning harmoniously together in delight over being at one with oneself, with others, and with the whole universe, has been distorted by negative emotional needs and the tyranny of the intellect.

Free and easy laughter is an expression of the basic simplicity and purity of spirit-dominated man who is not guilt-ridden, self-critical, or self-conscious. He does not even know what chronic anxiety is, but takes things as they come, relying on his own inner wisdom to direct his actions in daily life as well as on special occasions.

There are times when the spiritual psychotherapist may find himself stimulated to laugh in this natural manner by his unseen mentors in such a way that the patient also starts to laugh. I have seen such laughter be truly the best medicine for a depressed patient in mourning. There is nothing quite like it. Both patient and therapist are as if lifted into another sphere of being. The patient gets the feeling that he can, after all, surmount his difficulties much more easily than he thought and realises that a breakthrough has been made. Indeed it has been made by nothing more or less than highly infectious mirthful laughter in sheer delight.

Not every patient seen by the spiritual psychotherapist has caused a rupture between his lower and his higher self due to the stagnation which followed self-deception of a major degree. Nonetheless, he may be suffering from anxiety due to past conditioning. It may not serve any constructive purpose in such a case to work on factors pertaining to childhood. Dealing with present day matters in the presence of the therapist's own demonstration of positivity may be quite sufficient. The higher consciousness will direct a strong love force at the patient through the heart centre of the therapist, giving the patient the right kind of energy to find his way. It is astounding how valiantly some old souls have fought their way through a jungle of negativity and have yet retained a level of integrity. Of course, it is understood that such souls have received and accepted much fourth dimensional help, even if they have not been aware of it in their mortal consciousness.

Chapter 6

Psychopathology

The experience of pain removes objections in the personality to the governance of the Spirit. Letting go brings joy and well-being, regardless of outer circumstances. Dominance of the Spirit over the vehicle means one-ness, wholeness. This is a sensation which is strange and unaccustomed to civilised man who has hardly ever lived in harmony with his own nature and that surrounding him.

The higher Self of an "old" soul will stop short of nothing to cause its vehicle to subjugate itself, its thought, emotions, and activities to its rule. Every kind of misery, discomfort, sickness, every accident, every painful or disagreeable experience of any sort as well as every joy and exhilaration are designed to promote the dominance of the Spirit. The vehicle as such is of strictly temporary nature in all its aspects, serving only as a means, a valuable opportunity, for the higher Self to gather experience towards its maturation as an individuality with a depth and breadth of consciousness which the mortal mind on its own cannot grasp at all. The lesser cannot comprehend the greater, nor the mortal the eternal.

The overtrained and highly overestimated intellect of civilised man is often used as a defence against his own Spirit which is the life-giving principle itself. He is, thus, in the ridiculous position of biting the hand that feeds him. He need not then be surprised when that hand applies the discipline necessary to restore order and harmony, obedience to the master. This discipline hurts, even though it is truly executed in great love.

The spiritual psychotherapist must himself demonstrate wholeness or one-ness with his source. His state of simply BEING is as important for his patients as any words he may speak. He represents a sturdy rope or lifeline for those seeking to unify themselves, to consolidate their gains and steady their own being-ness in order to help others towards the same goal in their turn.

Nothing worthwhile is easy of attainment. An "old" soul does not expect a bed of roses in life. A student in the eighth year of school hardly expects to be given the same assignments and tests he was expected to complete in his second year. By the same token, however, he may look forward to deeper satisfactions, greater joys, and much more appreciation for the services he renders.

As long as man occupies a physical body he will be assailed by negativity in one or another form. It would be a pipe dream to believe that there would be no further pain and no more struggle when he has been cleared and is at one with himself. He will have to remain vigilant for as long as he is on earth. But with his Spirit in command of his thought and actions he will master all possible circumstances with poise and elegance, to the amazement of all who look to him for sustenance in their own struggle for at-one-ment.

Anyone who has worked within the confines of one of the established forms of psycho-analysis has been confronted with its limitations. Who doesn't know the story of patients in treatment for years without satisfactory results, not to speak of those who, less tenacious, drop out of treatment with at best very partial improvement in the quality of their living and being? I am certain that often these results are due to the fact that either the patient or the therapist or both, do not grasp the true meaning of life. Thus they narrow down their scope to the material and emotional circumstances and phantasies of the patient.

The "well-adjusted" individual often represents the goal of treatment. This implies a high degree of conformity with the expectations and mores of society, an adaptation to existing circumstances and conditions. No inquiry is made as to the Spirit's actual intent for the incarnation, what it wishes to accomplish. Well-adjusted conformity may not be its aim any more than senseless rebellion, or being different for the sake of being different. There is no substitute for individual man being true to himself, his real permanent Self. Real joy and satisfaction lie in the active striving for the genuine goal, whatever it may be. There is no uniformity of these aims, except that they all involve some deep inner progress of the individual soul, gained through the handling of living experience. Seen from the viewpoint of spiritual psychotherapy, what is normal and healthy in one case may well be pathological in another.

What the spiritual psychotherapist has to deal with most of all is negative conditioning. He has seen through and shed as much of his own as is humanly possible in order to be free to recognise that of his patients and to help them gain awareness of it. The amount of such negative conditioning varies in modern society from family to family and from individual to individual. At times it takes on grotesque forms. I shall cite just a few common instances of such conditioning, known to everyone: Being exposed to a draught is said to cause rheumatism or colds. The person imbued with such a notion will promptly get pain or a cold after sitting in a draught. One can, however, observe, that the same individual will be quite healthy after sitting in a boat in the wind. On both occasions there was simply air in motion. Yet I have been told by such people quite seriously that a draught and a wind are not at all the same thing, that only the former is dangerous, the latter being good for the constitution!

Another frequent conditioned thought concerns the drinking of alcoholic beverages. Due to the example set by adults, youngsters grow up associating this drinking with being grown up. Many feel they are not behaving as an adult if they do not participate in this habit.

Negative conditioning is the greatest stumbling block to individual unfoldment. Most damaging is the withholding from or rationing out to small children of the outward and visible signs of affection. The parent who herself or himself did not receive enough loving in early life very often finds it impossible to give real affection to the next generation. Indeed, parents are at times afraid they might do something wrong by being truly affectionate to the little ones. Withdrawal of affection is often used as a punishment for behaviour which does not meet adult specifications. These may appear senseless and unreasonable to small children and indeed are so at times. Discipline is a very poor substitute for love and yet there are parents who regard it as more important. If one were to put into one phrase the greatest difficulty of so-called civilised man today it would be: Not enough love.

Hatred, resentment, aggression, quarrelling, or lack of love in any form between the important adults in a child's life is picked up by the sensitive antennae of its awareness. When it is present or recurring over a long period of time it is applied to self and incorporated into the emotional pattern. In some cases the negative thinking and behaviour is imitated. When it cannot be imitated it may lead to an identity crisis later in life.

It is well-known in psychology that a child has the need to imitate the parent of the same sex and to a much lesser degree the other parent. When the parents, due to their own unresolved troubles, have not fulfilled their role as examples in a positive way, the child is damaged in turn. The more sensitive individual will generally be much more affected that the relatively sturdy, unimaginative one. For this reason, the former category is much more likely to require treatment than the latter.

The economic circumstances of the family during the childhood of patients are seldom of major importance in my experience. Even where some had gone hungry due to wartime deprivation, there was no associated damage to the personality if the adults in the child's environment had remained loving and calm during the experience. By contrast, I have noticed that among wealthy people the children, usually cared for by hired servants, have been exposed to varying degrees of deprivation of love and affection already in earliest infancy in a number of instances. In these cases the epitaph of the "poor little rich child" applies quite literally. Material riches cannot in any way make up for starving a child of the nourishment its soul needs; nor does poverty negate the value of true love.

Some patients have, in their young years, been exposed to emotional love and aggression alternately, so that they never knew what to expect from one day or one moment to the next. Such a child does not develop a relationship of normal trust with others later on. It is conditioned to be on guard defensively at all times.

Even when one or both parents had real love for the child, its expression can often be hampered, covered over, or distorted by faulty conditioning and disturbance in the parent's own emotionality and thought patterns. I have heard patients make statements such as these: "I'm not surprised my mother was that way, considering what her mother was like" or: "It's surprising my father wasn't even more messed up, considering how his father treated him".

The very many deficiencies and abnormalities in the love experiences of small children is very destructive to the feeling of self-worth. The little one who feels rejected, must needs form the idea that it is not lovable. When there has been constant reprimand and criticism, when honest effort has not been appreciated or praised, the child cannot develop any real self-assurance, nor any faith in its own ability, be it ever so outstanding.

Where self-confidence has never been properly supported the feelings are easily hurt. If the child's love for family members was rejected, it becomes afraid of showing or at times even feeling love for others. Behaviour may be aggressive without the patient actually being aware of it. Defence against real or imaginary attack is frequently expressed by aggression or withdrawal.

Fears of many forms and in many directions abound, They may be conscious or unconscious. The child which grows up in an environment which it does not understand is likely to try to find explanations by forming phantasies. These are often laden with emotions. When there is no real understanding from the adults, these phantasies may be repressed into the unconscious along with their accompanying emotions. That means they are forgotten. The trouble, however, is that they have not been eliminated but only "buried alive" where they are no longer available to be handled by adult reason at a later date. From their hidden recess they influence reactions, behaviour, and attitudes in any life situation, big or small, which even remotely or in some particle reminds the individual of the experiences leading up to the formation of the original phantasy. Once these phantasies have been brought into consciousness, together with their emotional content, the abnormal pattern promptly ceases to be. This sequence of events is well-known in standard depth-psychotherapy.

In spiritual psychotherapy there is the recognition that resentments, guilt feelings, attitudes, and characteristics are, at times, carry-overs from one or several previous incarnations. The soul which had not forgiven another in a previous lifetime may be embittered and resentful, accusing others of treating it wrongly. The patient may be quite aggressive in his behaviour and vengeful. As he hands out suffering he is very likely receiving it also. Usually he has no conscious awareness of the true origin of his trouble. He constitutes a hazard to those associated with him. Should such a one request treatment, it is essential that he be helped to remember the deed and person he had not forgiven. He may then recognise who, in his present life, is the soul of long ago. The act of forgiveness under these circumstances tends to have a most beneficial effect on both people, even in the other remains unaware of the past history.

The soul which has not forgiven itself for some crime or offence committed in a past experience tends to choose a harsh, punitive childhood environment and to continue the self-punitive pattern in some fashion. This can take many forms, even expressed in physical symptoms. Henry M. had for decades been suffering from recurrent severe pain in his spine above the waistline. Physical examinations and X-rays uncovered no abnormality which could account for it. Though this pain was not the reason why Henry M. came into spiritual psychotherapy, he at one point recollected a scene in one of the wars in ancient Greece in which he, as a warrior in battle, thrust his lance into the back of an enemy soldier at the same spot where the recurrent pain appeared. The dying soldier arched backward, so that his distorted features looked straight at the killer, who was horrified at his deed. Henry M. then exclaimed: "That was you! You were the victim!" He then consciously forgave himself for his "crime". I, the therapist, had no recollection of such an incarnation and said that if it was so, I felt no resentment. The back pains of Henry M. subsided thereafter. As far as I know they were gone within a few months. Maybe it took that long for his soul to forgive itself completely. After all, that is a very short time compared to the several thousand years during which this guilt feeling had been lodged in the soul.

I have repeatedly worked with patients who have remembered the salient features of other incarnations having a bearing on the present one to notice a consistent pattern. The soul chooses its new experiences in such a way that "undigested" parts of the pertinent former lives will be re-stimulated. This refers to character traits, attitudes, emotional habits, and thinking patterns acquired in other lives and not relinquished before leaving the body. These traits will then be brought to the fore in the present personality by the childhood environment and experiences in early life.

A woman, in a former life, had entered a convent voluntarily and, having made the customary vow of obedience, subjugated herself to the unreasonable discipline demanded by the religious order and the Mother Superior, thereby subordinating herself to the tyranny of younger souls despite the warnings of the "still small voice" within.

This patient, in the present life, was raised by parents who made hard disciplinary requirements which were often quite unnatural. The many prohibitions and demands thus instilled in the child made for much emotional suffering and hardships in adult life. This eventually led to a search for enlightenment and to a desperate inner call for help which paved the way for being guided to the mediator and thence to the spiritual psychotherapist. The difficulties were overcome. The individual would ever after be careful not to submit to the tyranny of a younger soul, but walk upright and self-confident through life, obedient only to the higher Self.

In several instances I have had patients who had spent an incarnation in some monastery, remote from ordinary life, in one instance, even haughtily looking down upon natural sexuality. These people have, in their present lives, had childhood experiences designed to stimulate a variety of extra-ordinary sexual expressions. In this case there was mixed hetero- and homosexuality that continued into adult years. This person, who had previously looked askance at sexual activities is a man in this incarnation with experience of great promiscuity in his young years leading to venereal infections on several occasions. When these men and women come for help, often for a reason not consciously related to their sexual problems, they have a fine opportunity to come to terms with the past and present extremes in their attitudes and behaviour, having uncovered the cause. How much work is to be done in the individual case on the roots of difficulties in the present life before uncovering or detailing related former incarnations is best left to the therapist's skilled inspirers who are cognisant of the needs of the particular person.

There are patients whose childhood environment and relationship with the important adults were such that the personality cannot get onto a firm basis even after emotional matters have been brought into the open. This happens especially when the adult example was so poor that the child had no-one to identify with. Conventional treatment then can lead to a relative adjustment but that is not a truly fulfilling life. Such a patient may not be able to accept the positivity radiated at him. The unseen experts have on occasion been able to revive in such a one the memory of another incarnation in which he grew up with loving parents and in full knowledge of the one-ness of man and nature. There is no hypnosis used in this process ever. Once the memory is present the patient is told to hold the scene in which he finds himself, reliving the sensation of love and affection. This opens his receptivity to love energy in the present time and gives him at least some positive identification on which to build. Even one such experience has a most salutary effect, but the patient can then also use the memory at will again to steady himself more.

In several such instances, which I recall, the patients were taken back into incarnations as North American Indians of times long past. These people knew the Great Spirit to be the indivisible totality and their own spirit as part of it. One young man experienced himself as an Indian toddler being picked up and held by his strong and loving father and feeling the peace, security and deep affection. The same entity who was, at that remote time, his bodily father spoke to him through a mediator, simultaneously reinforcing the patient's identification with the feeling of positivity and self-worth in the other incarnation.

I have marvelled at the effectiveness of this technique in instances in which I, personally, could not see where the necessary "props" could come from to give the personality a really solid foundation. The reader should take note that the support was not obtained by identification with a life in which a high social station, fame, or fortune was given, but with a state of being and feeling, of loving and being loved, of joy and security, of one-ness with nature and God. These are real values which can be brought through into the present and, as it were, reawakened. That is the purpose of this new method. It has no interest in supplying the means for developing conceit over having been some "important" personage once upon a time.

So-called civilised man has created conditions which predispose individuals to self-abnegation, usually because of a fear or fears super-imposed on an already damaged personality. A betrayal of self has a devastating effect on man's wholeness. The higher and lower selves normally function as a unit, like a cowboy and his horse. He loves his animal, takes fine care of it night and day. The horse thrives and is content, feeling secure under his guidance and guardianship. Self-betrayal is equivalent to the horse bucking and kicking, trying to get away from the cowboy or throwing him off, so that he's just holding on by the bridle. Naturally, he will do all he can to gain control over the horse again. Injury may occur to either one or both in the process.

The lower self, the personality, suffers greatly in such a condition, not only emotionally but often also physically and through myriad "outer" circumstances brought about by itself even though they appear to be caused by others. Various degrees of states of stagnation are thus generated. At times, the afflicted individuals give the impression of being embroiled in an internal civil war which they also manage to externalise, at least in part.

A therapist familiar with this condition is constantly amazed at the frequency of its occurrence. It is given various classical diagnoses, depending on the way it happens to show itself in a given instance. The spiritual psychotherapist is much less concerned about a usual diagnosis than he is about establishing peace between the warring camps as rapidly as possible. The results of re-established harmony are most gratifying indeed, often astounding.

The undermining of self-esteem for a long time, either in childhood or in adult life, is a most serious problem. Being seriously criticised, "put down", or put on the defensive by repeated accusations causes the recipient of such treatment to lose spontaneity of action. This spontaneity, or just being, is of very major importance in the normal healthy person. Natural unselfconsciousness gives way to self-observation, self-criticism and self-justification. Fearfulness and other destructive tendencies develop. Thinking at times takes the place of doing as the personality takes refuge in it.

In families in which the adults demonstrate the "stiff upper lip" kind of emotional repression, the young also grow up to be fearful of their own emotions, of being natural. At times they believe they actually don't have strong emotions. This leads to peculiar reaction patterns. Until such people are freed from their conditioning, their life pattern cannot properly unfold.

Another common mechanism in Western culture is the notion that sexuality and sexual expression is separate from other aspects of living. False teachings and indoctrination have added considerably to this burden. The resultant abnormalities are very common and quite varied. Spiritual psychotherapy sees and treats them from the viewpoint of a wide-angle lens, as part of the total consciousness rather than in a separate compartment.

At times a patient adheres to a habitual thinking pattern even after its roots have been uncovered. This happens primarily when the habit was well established in one or more other incarnations and then re-stimulated in the present one. The therapist must then advise the patient how he can overcome the pattern and re-channel the energies into constructive pathways. Where rebellion has been a major part of the trouble, the patient may have quite a battle on his hands. The therapist will need patience and a good sense of humour. If he remains positive the victory is assured. One or two little exercises, geared to the individual patient, will teach him to let the higher Self establish a firm hold on the outer personality. The therapist will receive all the necessary help from the higher dimension and may become aware of considerable amusement in these ranks at the last desperate struggles of the little ego to forestall its inevitable surrender to its one and only Reality.

Compassionate unemotional understanding is the basis for all spiritual psychotherapy, regardless of the approach. The depth of the understanding will vary with the knowledge and experience of the therapist and with the degree of acceptance he demonstrates for what he is taught by his skilled mentors on the higher dimensional level.

Some "old" souls have a deep grasp of karmic processes which penetrates into the mortal consciousness. For very deep and varied therapy such a comprehensive understanding is of the essence, as it can be stimulated and used by the unseen experts impinging upon the thought of the therapist. The need for such experienced souls in incarnation to do the work of "clearing out" is great. The number of individuals ready to be "cleared out" is rapidly increasing.

According to reliable higher dimensional sources the rescue of this planet from the destructive madness of its inhabitants depends on the number of "old" souls in incarnation who, having recognised themselves as souls, undergo the process of clearance so that their heart and brow centres (these are also known as chakras or energy vortices) can be used for the transmission of positive energies in their pure state into the collective consciousness of the human beings within the orbit of each.

" I GIVE UNTO YOU A PATH AND A WAY"

Section II

The Work in Action

Chapter 7

When a Child is Born

A child at birth has already been on earth for nine months; its spirit has been, if not actually in its body the whole time, then at least intimately associated with it. Having chosen its parents from its original dimension, it is then exposed to their state of being and takes part in their circumstances, happenings, emotions and thoughts all the time its body is being fashioned in the mother's womb.

All life is thought. The spirit or soul comes from a far greater consciousness than it will ever experience while it is on earth. Coming into its new incarnation it loses its great awareness and with it the sense of its true identity. The process may be likened to the turning of a dimmer switch from maximum to minimum wattage. The earthly waking consciousness, then, is like the bit of an iceberg which shows above the water level. The larger subconscious and unconscious is out of sight. The unborn, is, however, acutely sensitive, can see, sense and hear from the start, long before its physical sense organs and its nervous system are formed and finished.

The true nature of the soul is love. It expects to be loved by its parents. It needs to be welcomed and enjoyed by loving parents already as a pregnancy. This joy creates in the newcomer a positive attitude and feeling toward self from the start. A natural people like the North American Indians of old times felt that every baby was a gift from the Great Spirit, to be revered by all.

A child conceived and carried in such an atmosphere has no doubt about its own value. It looks forward eagerly to its sojourn on earth and is a picture of peace and contentment from birth. Its parents will have been emotionally mature adults, calm, cheerful and harmonious, together enjoying their creative task of supplying the body for an incoming soul.

Eons of evolution have conditioned man and beast alike to need this free flow of love and enjoyment for normal development. It is a matter of a deep abiding feeling. For the incoming soul it is a necessity, not a luxury, if a positive self-image is to develop. Love is the food for the soul while the body is being fed by physical matter, so it can grow and develop.

There is an inexhaustible supply of love from the spirit when no barrier has been erected to impede its flow. Emotions, on the other hand, are of the earth. They are an integral part of the make-up of the physical body, involving the secretions from endocrine (ductless) glands, mediated by and through the autonomic (involuntary) nervous system, i.e. the sympathetic and parasympathetic systems. The common expression, "the adrenaline is flowing" indicates some popular awareness of these facts in the twentieth century.

When people are in harmony with themselves and each other the spirit, the eternal self, is in control of the entire physical mechanism, like a good driver is of his car. The spirit needs the emotional part of the body machine to express itself and function on the material level. So, while the spirit is in charge, all is well. However if the spirit (or soul) is held at bay, prevented from taking the controls, love does not flow and emotion predominates. The foetus cannot make do with purely emotional "love" which is short-lived or up and down by its very nature. It is more confusing and unsettling than reassuring.

Basic to all real love is the love of self, self being the mortal and the immortal being as a functioning unit. Compare this arrangement to a rider in old times who needed to go places. He had to be able to rely on his horse. A relationship of trust between rider and horse was essential. The two could never be the same, but together they had to function as a unit, the horse responding without hesitation to the rider's touch as the rider responded to the horse's needs. The two had to be friends to achieve optimum functioning.

When the parents are at one, each with himself or herself and with each other, the little one is fine with itself and them from the very start. Nature has it that the basic feeling attitude toward self is forged at this early stage of an incarnation. There is nothing anyone can do about this fact. It is natural law.

After birth the baby needs to be held by mother, be put to the breast. Being on mother's body it continues to feel her breathing movements, even to hear her heart beat, as well as her now unmuffled voice. Again, it needs to be warmly welcomed and enjoyed physically, emotionally and spiritually by both its parents. For entirely normal development, human beings, like some of their animal cousins, need to be bonded with both parents and raised by them. Real bonding is genuine tender love which the little one amply returns in kind, very, very early.

Although the pre-natal, natal and post-natal child has a feeling attitude about itself from taking on board the parents' thoughts about it, it does not yet have a proper sense of identity. In fact, a great deal of loving handling, stroking and patting, which stimulate the sensory nerve receptors, first give it the feeling of inhabiting its own skin, its own space. Animal mothers to a large extent produce the same effect in their young by licking them tenderly. Monkeys and apes use their hands much as man.

Though the little one has already been conditioned through its environment by the time it is born, very intensive conditioning takes place afterwards. Much of this is determined by cultural factors then as well as by the parents' own personal pattern, as the parents themselves were conditioned already as little ones. This causes the often very different collective personalities of groupings or even whole nations. Where love, and therefore self-esteem, prevails, these differences are of no danger, but add welcome variety and colour to the society.

Human beings, by their very nature, do not automatically grow up into emotionally, spiritually and socially adult individuals independently as some creatures do. They are, from start to finish of their long growing period, dependent on role models. I often say that we are "monkey see, monkey do", and this for better or for worse.

Each child will normally try to copy primarily the parent of the same sex as it is encouraged to do by the adults. However, its relationship with the parent of the opposite sex is almost more important still to its later adult behaviour and self-image.

If the parents are essentially grown-up within themselves and loving each other, all is well. The parent of the same sex will present the little one with an image of positivity accepted within the culture, an example which the child can safely imitate until it has adopted the pattern as its own. Simultaneously, the parent of the opposite sex will encourage the offspring in this imitation. All these things will take place in play and fun and with plenty of laughter under healthy conditions, quite naturally and easily. Who has not seen little girls playing hard at being little women and boys at being men, imitating their elders? As they get older and more outward-turned, they add other role models, When the atmosphere at home has been a loving and harmonious one, they will tend to veer towards positive models outside the home, becoming solid and constructive citizens of their respective societies.

Chapter 7.1 - Agoraphobia

Jane panicked whenever she left home and found herself in a public place. There were times when she had to use a suburban railway to go to a neighbouring town. Coming out of the station which faced a busy street, Jane found herself so terrified, with heart pounding, hands sweating and breathing fast and shallow, that she felt everyone could see her state. She would run back into the station and take the next train home, leaving all her errands undone.

The condition became worse. Jane could not go out to work anymore, was rarely able to do her shopping. She was tied to her house like an invalid and very unhappy. Her husband, she felt, must be very tired of the situation, so that she began to fear for her marriage.

Jane had a real love and flair for interior decorating. She was artistic in a number of ways. She would have liked to establish herself doing business along these lines, but know she could not as long as her severely neurotic condition paralysed every effort to reach out and deal with the public.

She had already tried several ways of getting help: psychotherapy, hypnotherapy, and tranquillisers from her family doctor. None had helped for more than a short time and the drugs made her feel like a zombie.

In her despair she came to see us as a "last resort". It emerged immediately that her mother had always considered her own marriage as a mistake. She had had an unfortunate love affair and on the rebound had started another affair with Jane's father right after. A pregnancy resulted and the two got married quickly. That baby miscarried after the wedding, but the couple stayed together. Jane was the next pregnancy in this mismatch between two people, neither of whom was truly grown up or knew what love really is. Little Jane was perceived by her mother as a final seal on the unhappy union. Being incapable of loving under those circumstances, neither parent could bond with the little one before or after birth. Mother did her best, caring for Jane and later children conscientiously, and father was an equally dutiful provider. Yet there was no joy in the family life, little laughter, and much self-sacrificing by mother.

At no time could little Jane feel really good about herself. Self-esteem could not develop. Fears and apprehensions were her constant companions. Away from home she saw children and adults who seemed unselfconscious and enjoying themselves. How she envied their bliss!

It was easy for Jane to understand that her unbonded state and the joyless upbringing led to her persistent feelings of vulnerability. However, this realisation was not sufficient to free her from her symptoms of agoraphobia (fear of open or public places). She needed to know why her soul had chosen her particular childhood environment. To that end she had to discover what she had been and done in some other life-times.

There had, indeed, been several life-times in which she had given in to fear and anger, wilfully escaping into protected settings rather than taking her chances with ordinary living. Twice, at least, she had chosen to enter a monastery or convent, closing the door behind herself. In the life before the present one she had incarnated as a girl into a Muslim society in which women were considered of less value than a camel. She was married off young to a man she did not know, who put her into his harem. There she was shut away from all opportunity to express herself freely and constructively.

In the Muslim life she had had no choice of action and no rights. As the soul had not used its opportunities in several previous lives, it had then chosen to take an incarnation in which it hit bottom to an extent that was designed to do away with the previously persistent willfulness so that progress could be resumed afterwards.

The method had worked. Despite fear and anger, Jane was not rebellious. Once more in a free Western society, the soul now had the opportunity to overcome infantile fear and rage and to fulfil itself.

Jane realised that there was no point in trying to identify with members of her family or in expecting her loving, patient husband to make up to her what she had missed out on as a baby. She had to stop perceiving her own soul as she had experienced her parents as a child, as letting her down in their ineptness.

To help her identify with her spirit we did a little exercise with her, during which she actively felt her own true reality. This proved to be an unforgettable experience for her. She could repeat the technique at will as often as she pleased, and it would make it progressively easier for the immature child in her to form a self-image of real adulthood, feeling the love, strength and joy of her immortal soul.

Jane was quickly aware that this identification would bring laughter, enjoyment and enterprise into her daily life. Fear would soon evaporate. Her creative talent would find expression in a self-confident, professional way.

We did go into Jane's dietary pattern with her. Her physical body was entitled to maximum vigour. She had had trouble trouble with soft, thin, peeling fingernails and from time to time periods of easy bruising. These were a sure sign of a marked Vitamin D deficiency. We asked her to take a one-a-day capsule of cod liver oil regularly for as long as she was living in this far northern climate. The deficiency of this particular vitamin had definitely increased her anxiety state, and made it more difficult for her to come to grips with her emotions.

Jane needed to see us twice more in two years as she went up and down a bit. But then she levelled off. She has every right to feel proud of herself. Having overcome the fear and anguish of several successive life-times she is now truly an example of positive achievement for all the people who know and meet her.

Chapter 7.2 - Puzzling Actions of Babies and Small Children

A young couple had a two-year old son who, from birth, had obviously preferred his father to his mother. He seemed invariably thrilled when father held him, spoke with him or played with him. Then a girl was born. This little one was delighted from the beginning when in the presence of her mother, but, even in the newborn stage, she consistently turned her face away from her father as soon as he entered the room. She made her feelings abundantly clear. When she had behaved in this fashion for weeks, the father wailed "I do believe she doesn't like me!". The child was about one and a half years old when she surprised herself by wanting contact with Dad. Once she had climbed on his lap by her own volition, the ice was broken and she never fell back into the old stance.

The story remained a puzzle in the family until Soul Directed Therapy uncovered the fact that a deep-seated resentment had remained in the girl from another life in which she had been the daughter of the same soul as father. At that time he had treated her and her mother most shabbily, banning both of them from his presence and from their home community because he wanted a younger woman who might bear him a son. The elder brother's experience had been a very different one in that same past life-time. He had, indeed, been the coveted son born to that father later in life by a second wife.

A similar case is that of Rita. She was the premature baby of an unmarried woman who died in childbirth. As the grandmother had to work, she put the child into an orphanage. At three months of age the baby was adopted by a childless and loving couple.

Whenever the adoptive mother tried to cuddle and kiss her, the little one turned and struggled away. However, when a neighbouring woman came in, the baby was most affectionate and responsive to her. Rita grew up still keeping herself aloof from mother.

Soul Directed Therapy uncovered a life-time long ago in which the adoptive mother had been a judge who sentenced a man to death. The man felt unjustly convicted and died with a deep resentment against the judge. The soul of the convict had now reincarnated as the premature girl baby whose life was saved by the loving tender care of the judge's soul, incarnated this time as the adoptive mother. The girl's soul has been given a chance to overcome that deep resentment. The mother's soul took the opportunity to save an incarnation where the judge had previously destroyed one, thus repaying the old debt.

Chapter 8

What is the Body?

Bodies are matter. What we call matter is made up of molecules which consist of atoms which in turn consist of sub-atomic "particles". On that level the distinction as we perceive it between matter and energy or non-matter ceases to exist.

I remember how I felt when I first realised that, from the viewpoint of physics, if the space between the atoms constituting a human body were removed, all the atoms would fit into the head of a pin. This would be the case if the atoms themselves were solid, which they are not.

I never studied nuclear physics. Yet enough of its findings have been published in easily comprehensible form to point up the unreality of matter. I liken it to the order of reality of an image on a motion picture screen which is not the thing itself or the actors in person but convincingly real to the viewer when he is absorbed in the action depicted and identifies with the characters for the duration due to "the willing suspension of disbelief".

The body is subject to the natural law of earth. To function efficiently as the earthly vehicle of the spirit it must be fed according to its needs. Just as different species of animals have different food requirements, different races of man are not quite alike either. Neither are all the individuals within a given or mixed racial grouping.

Common sense dictates that each body must be fed according to its genetic constitution, which will be evident in a number of ways, and not according to somebody's moralistic thinking and indoctrination. With some of the ideas coursing around in and out of print in this respect, one can only say that "the road to hell is paved with good intentions".

It is quite evident that, in many circumstances, if the farmer or breeder fed his livestock as carelessly as he feeds himself or his family, he would not be able to bring his animals to market.

A pristine spirit, with all its wisdom, can hardly be expected to be able to keep control over a body whose brain, peripheral and autonomic nervous systems cannot function correctly because of faulty nutrition, and whose stress system, which includes the endocrine glands, has one bombshell after another thrown at it by way of gross nutritional poisons and imbalances.

Truly valuing the body and caring for it inside and out is tantamount to the love of the spirit self. This also applies to the way a person appears in public, how neatly and attractively dressed and presented. Nobody can possibly believe that the individual who runs around in drab, ugly or ungainly clothing and hair-styles demonstrates any measure of self-respect. Dignity in all things is a very important component of the love of self. A person who does not show self-esteem cannot be trusted to value others and cannot, therefore, expect to be respected by them. In the words of Abraham Lincoln's Gettysburgh Address: "You can fool some of the people some of the time; but you cannot fool all the people all the time".

Above all, one cannot fool the spirit. It sees the truth, always.

Given proper nutrition and care, the state of the body, especially its health, is intimately related to the emotional balance or the lack of it and to the state of the soul itself.

All dis-ease comes from the soul, without exception. Even accidents are only apparently accidental. The eternal law of course and effect makes no mistake.

As the entire universe is thought, right thinking causes good health and a state of well-being. Wrong thinking, which includes deleterious attitudes brings symptoms in the body, disease, injuries or even self-destruction when the individual concerned will not change.

As the body is itself consciousness it is easy to see why it is so responsive to thought, both positive and negative. It is equally obvious why, despite modern scientific medicine, the incidence of chronic degenerative diseases has increased rather than decreased in industrialised countries, no doubt parallel to the loss of simplicity in thinking and being, and to the decline of love given to little ones.

Chapter 8.1 - Food and Drink

It is to be remembered that dietary patterns, both food and drink, are very important constituents of cultural patterns everywhere. The old statement "Mens sana in corpore sano", a healthy mind in a healthy body, is as true today as it ever was. Food and drink have a profound effect on physical, emotional, mental and spiritual well-being as people find out when they change from an unsound nutritional pattern to a sensible one and vice versa. When the food or drink habit is a deleterious one, I liken the situation to a driver trying to drive a car containing the wrong petrol or a rider trying to control an ill-fed horse.

It is also essential to realise that different racial groups have different nutritional requirements. Did not the physical ancestry of various races live long ago in different climatic conditions with varying food supplies? In our society today there are many conflicting idea systems abroad regarding diet. For the most part, no account is taken of differences of requirements from person to person, often on the basis of heredity. The cacophony of voices is confusing to those who do not have a firmly-founded scientific background knowledge.

For instance, in my practice I have seen many people who were obviously in an iron-deficiency anaemia because they were not eating meat when they were of the genetic type which cannot absorb iron from plant sources.

Very often in recent years, I have encountered people in more or less profound salt deficiency states because they have taken the anti-salt propaganda too seriously, and are themselves of a physical constitution which needs a steady and adequate supply of salt. When these people consult me, I give them a salty drink which, within minutes, improves their looks, gives them a sense of well-being and enables their brain to function properly. It is a fact that salt deficiency causes oedœma (swelling) of the brain. We have heard of such statements as: "Oh, I feel as if I've just woken up", or "I'm suddenly with it".

When it comes to nutritional poisons like alcohol, people do not realise that, although the liver removes the alcohol from the blood stream in at most half a day, there has been much more lasting damage done to the membranes of the brain cells. These consist of a very thin layer of a lipid (fat-like) substance which dissolves in a powerful fat-solvent like alcohol. Repairing these membranes of the surviving cells takes from two to seven days, depending on the quantity of intake. However, we have seen people who felt that their finer brain functions required a much longer period for full restoration. The killed-off brain cells can never be replaced.

Besides the effect on the nervous system, these substances derange the smooth functioning of the stress mechanism of which the adrenal cortical glands are a very essential part. I have often compared the stress mechanism to a symphony orchestra playing beautiful music. When harsh nutritional poisons, like alcohol, caffeine or quantities of sugar are consumed, they act like hand grenades thrown into the orchestra pit. If then one expects the orchestra to produce fine music again in a short time, this demand is quite unrealistic. It takes time to repair the damage and reconstitute order. More often than not the next bomb is already arriving before the shambles from the previous one has been repaired.

I once asked a woman who was fond of a glass or two of wine with her dinner how she would like to ride a horse which had partaken of a small amount of an alcoholic beverage. She became quite agitated as she exclaimed: "No way! I wouldn't touch it. I am an experienced horsewoman". It was then easy for me to point out to her that she was expecting her experienced rider, her own God-self, to be able to control and direct her alcohol-damaged body, mind and emotions efficiently and creatively. I knew she would never feel comfortably complacent about her drinking again.

The contents of tobacco smoke are also classed among nutritional poisons for obvious reasons. How often have I seen people greatly concerned with various faddy nutritional ideas of which they understood little while continuing to load their precious bodies with the great variety of poisons in tobacco smoke. It contains not only nicotine but also extremely toxic substances like the metal cadmium and carbon monoxide. Where is the common sense? It is the most uncommon sense of all.

Chapter 8.2 - M.E.

Carol came to see us recently because she had been unable to work for the last three years at her job as stockbroker. She had had a short succession of virus infections followed by what had been diagnosed as "M.E.", post-viral encephalopathy.

Carol knew that she had always had a low blood pressure. It was easy to assure her that this was very common, not at all abnormal and in no way dangerous to life and health. Had any professional ever told her how she could "live happily ever after" with this hereditary pattern? No. She had been advised not to eat much meat. She had never added much salt to her food. In fact, for years she had not paid much attention to what she ate, doing it the easy way. Breakfast, lunch and tea-time snack consisted almost entirely of carbohydrates, namely, cereals, flour and sugar. Dinner was more sensible, but generally contained potatoes in some form. Potato starch is quite rapidly converted into glucose in the small intestine.

It was explained to Carol that the sudden absorption of large amounts of glucose into the blood stream constituted attacks on her stress mechanism. A sudden rise in blood sugar is an emergency. If the glucose level remains high, this would be diabetes. Therefore, the liver must be caused to remove the extra sugar from the blood quickly, converting it into glycogen which is stored mainly in the liver for future measured reconversion into glucose and/or deposition as fat.

With her low blood pressure, Carol has a stress system which is even more sensitive to the sugar onslaught than that of other physiological types. Normally the endocrine or ductless glands which regulate the blood sugar function like a symphony orchestra playing harmonious music. The nutritional attacks have an effect like hand grenades thrown into the orchestra pit, exploding here and there. Before repairs have been completed, the next grenade has already arrived.

A shambles of any sort within the stress system will make the maintenance of a sense of well-being and robust health quite impossible. In addition to her high intake of the wrong kinds and quantities of sugary and starchy foods, Carol was also getting too little salt for her physiological type which lets go of salt quickly via the kidneys and therefore needs constant and adequate replacement. Salt is a necessity for the body, not a luxury. Of course, it is to be remembered that not everyone is of Carol's kind and that there are some who tend to hold salt rather than excreting it. Carol's type, running around in a salt deficiency, feels this as a state of listlessness, weakness, fatigue, the nearest thing to depression.

We gave Carol a lukewarm cup of salty broth while she was with us. About ten minutes later we could see a marked change in her features and she was very aware of a sudden shift in her state of being. She said "Oh, I feel like I just woke up!" The world looked quite different to her. I explained that the salt deficiency had caused some swelling of her brain which was, in that state, quite unable to function well.

I had given her a hand mirror and asked her to memorise her features, their form and colour, just before she drank the broth. Then, when she had "woken up", I asked her to look again. She had no trouble describing the differences which included shining eyes. Her eyes had previously been rather dull. The salt deficiency had also caused some swelling in the facial tissues which were now normalised, making her look years younger and also prettier.

As Carol now had a lively intelligence, we were able to proceed apace with other matters. That intelligence is actually of the spirit which was now able to use its earthly vehicle to advantage. Its relief and joy about the change shone out all over Carol. She felt ready to tackle life with gusto, making up for lost time.

Chapter 8.3 - Anorexia and Bulimia

Kathy's mother lived alone with her three children, aged fourteen, twelve and nine, after her husband left her for another woman. He had been difficult, at times even violent; yet, understanding his very deprived childhood, the wife had loved him and now felt abandoned and betrayed. In her undermined state she was ready to grasp at straws.

A considerably younger man whom she met was attracted to her, and she started an affair with him. Within a few months, she realised she was pregnant. He was not unhappy about it, but the lady did not, could not, really love him, and refused to marry him. The child born from this affair was Kathy. The mother felt trapped in the situation. When Kathy was about two years old, her mother married the young man for the child's sake.

The older children, deeply disturbed by their father's departure and their mother's undermined state, saw little Kathy as a most unwelcome intruder, and made her feel that she was an outsider as she had a different Daddy.

The child grew up feeling isolated and unloved, much like Cinderella. Nothing she did in order to win recognition or approval ever succeeded. She became quite withdrawn.

When Kathy was twelve years old, her parents separated. The older children were no longer at home. Mother and daughter then lived alone together in a joyless way. At fourteen years of age Kathy developed anorexia nervosa and bulimia. She had always been slightly overweight, but at fourteen she disliked her looks intensely and saw herself as an ugly duckling. She was in fact a rather pretty girl. She went through periods of not eating alternating with over-eating and then making herself vomit. There was the idea that dieting would make her more attractive, more likable: " I felt there was something not right about me. My periods of near-starvation, then over eating and vomiting became more and more uncontrollable, in fact compulsive. Try as I would, I couldn't master myself. The worse I became, the more fed-up and disgusted with me my mother became. I developed strong guilt feelings about it all. I alternated between fear and downright despair."

Kathy had always been a conscientious pupil, a high achiever in school. Now, while continuing with her scholastic achievement, she also became quite over-active in sports, feeling that this would make her more acceptable. She made herself believe that she enjoyed all the excessive running and competing. It was really a self-punishing way of trying to find her identity in the world.

At sixteen, a desperate Kathy ran away from home. She went to London to stay with a friend. Her symptoms improved considerably for a while, but the other girl found Kathy altogether too difficult and decided she could not bear her any longer. The mere thought of going back to mother made Kathy very ill. In her despair, she made up her mind to be a prostitute. She was picked up by a man who had never picked up a girl before. He acted on a sudden impulse. A good and decent human being, he saw through Kathy's desperation and recognised her intrinsic value. He took her in and looked after her.

While searching for some professional help for her, he found out about our work. Kathy was more than willing to be helped by this time, and her benefactor was ready to pay our fee for her treatment.

With our help, Kathy saw quite easily why she would have felt herself to be a calamity from the time her mother discovered the unwanted pregnancy. She understood that she had never experienced love until she was taken in hand by the man who had picked her up and truly cared for her. Kathy had never known what it is to feel good about oneself, to have self-esteem.

We recognised her as an "old" soul, one with many earth lives behind her, with great ability and the innate wisdom of long experience.

Besides a clear look at the elements which had shaped her personality in the present life so far, the medium was able to inform Kathy of the two incarnations just preceding, which had much to do with her choice of the particular home situation to which she had subjected herself this time round.

Two life-times back, Kathy had been in charge of an orphanage and been responsible for hard and harsh treatment meted out to the unhappy children in her care. They had experienced no love from her or her staff. Wishing to redress the sadistic tendency exercised at that time, the soul next chose a life in which, again as a woman, she became a hospital nurse. Underpaid and over-worked, she lived a life of self-sacrifice and suffering.

Hearing this, Kathy said: "No wonder I've always said that the last thing I wanted to be is a nurse. I had enough of being one the last time!"

We explained to Kathy that her recent lives had been all about learning the lesson of love, giving it and receiving it in an easy, spontaneous flow in daily life and doings. Her eternal Self knew that in the present life it could overcome all the damage done to the personality in its growing years. The deprived, fearful, angry and rebellious little girl still operating in the grown-up body could be taught, gently but firmly, to stop equating the magnificent true self with the undermined, loveless personalities of the earthly parents. All that was needed was that the temporary self make friends with the permanent self and learn to trust it as it had never been able to trust the parents and older brothers and sisters.

After the session with us, Kathy walked out on air. Life would never be the same again. In a short time she discovered a great interest in astrology and studied it in depth. Her fine intelligence and perceptiveness helped her in this pursuit.

Eventually, she set herself up in the professional practice of astrology. She was able to bring the experience of her own suffering to her sessions. Soon she realised she was also helping her clients with her psychic gifts.

Her practice is flourishing by this time, as she is giving excellent treatment which frees people from past-life residues and childhood traumas.

Cinderella has become the Queen.

Chapter 9

Sensing

The human consciousness is comparable to a television set. No-one would claim that the machine is the originator or the sender of the programs. It is simply a receiver. What it receives and communicates will invariably depend on the channel to which it is tuned.

Man's perception has two possibilities. That means he is capable of sensing on one of two levels:

> a) the intellectual level;
> b) the intuitive level.

Many people live totally on the intellectual level, either being unaware that there is another one or refusing to give it recognition. Much energy is wasted by those who keep trying to divine what the spirit has to say while they wilfully remain on the lower, intellectual/emotional level of understanding.

The difficulty basically arises in the very earliest part of the life. Lack of parental bonding pre- and post-natally makes it almost impossible for an individual thereafter to distinguish the true Self from the earthly personality. The early deprivation causes people to go through life still full of their need for love. They do not realise that "needing" of this sort is utterly infantile. Feeling needy, they are unable to harmonise with their own spirit because of the anger, almost hate, which they carry in the personality. Subconsciously they are continuously attacking the Self, running it down and in no way appreciating it.

There is, then, a terrific conflict between the inner infant and the authority of Self. The infant is not prepared to accept this authority in any way. In this fashion, such people gradually ruin their lives by living on the material level only. Their total lack of fulfilment creates symptoms in the body and often also actual physical disease.

The antipathy toward what is sensed or perceived as the authority of the soul is actually the deprived or rejected infant's anger, rebellion and resentment against the "delinquent" or "treacherous" adults on whom it was totally dependent for a long, long time. The picture is that of a NO TRUST situation.

Liken the personality to a horse which has been neglected and mistreated by its handler. Along comes a new handler. He or she cannot do a thing with the horse unless trust can be established. The new handler is suspected of being as unreliable, negligent or cruel as the former one was experienced to be. The new master sets out to prove his or her love and tenderness to the horse. If conversion does not succeed, the two can never function as a harmonious team enjoying each other's company in work and play, indeed functioning as one.

This parable has helped many to begin to find the way out of their dilemma.

Chapter 10

Whys and Wherefores

The human intellect can only partially comprehend how the law of cause and effect determines our living experience.

A more profound understanding requires the deep realisation that earth life is not at all what it appears to be as seen through the myopic lens of the material consciousness.

Man cannot change the law of cause and effect one iota. It is supremely and unalterably operative in all things at all times. Its perfect design gives every soul endless opportunity to learn what truth is.

To people who are capable of seeing through appearances and grasping origins, it is plain that all illnesses, all symptoms, even all accidents, are psychosomatic in nature, without a single exception. An inspired investigation into their cause will quickly illumine the origin in the present life and/or one or more past lives of the stricken individual. Equally obvious will be the purpose of the experience in the soul's learning pattern.

Some examples will help to make these few statements more transparent.

Chapter 10.2 - Broken Bones

Sara had been an unbonded child with several years of emotional trauma experienced during a war situation. Her self-image had remained essentially that of a vulnerable, hurt child. She was married to a truly loving man who was not able to alter this basic misconception of hers. Sara had many strong guilt feelings which she could not verbalise well. Her intense fears and anger had always been a problem but she was a very strong character. When she was in her forties her husband's beloved aunt died. Within three months of this event both of Sara's parents died in her own house. Sara had nursed them, one after the other, with the help of her husband when he was not out working.

Following the third passing, her mother's, Sara was so frantic that the family doctor advised her husband to hire someone to stay with her while he was at work and the children at school. A young woman was quickly found. She could come in for a few weeks. Sara was washing her hands in the bathroom a few days after her mother's death when she clearly heard her mother's voice in her head: "Take off your rings! Your fingers are going to swell." Sara slid the rings off and placed them on the glass shelf over the basin. Before she could dry her hands, she heard the signal of an arriving delivery van in front of the house. She hurried out of the front door, then slipped on a tiny spot of ice on the front path, falling headlong. She suffered a displaced fracture of her left wrist and forearm. The pain was tremendous.

The bones were set under anaesthesia, the hand and arm casted. The usual prolonged period of healing and after-care followed. Sara's attention was most effectively diverted from her excessive grief and rage onto her fracture. She felt later that the accident had saved her sanity at the time and she was grateful that her lovely rings had not had to be cut from her swollen fingers.

Chapter 10.3 - Despair

Peggy was an only child. Her parents cared for her but were unable to bond with her as they themselves had not been bonded, and thus had never learned what love is. They were quite rich. Peggy could have whatever she wanted materially and socially, but not true love.

A grandmother lived not very far away. She took the place of a positive mother as much as she could as Peggy spent much time in her house, especially during holidays. Feeling Grandmother's warm interest, Peggy learned to communicate with her freely, unloading all her little sorrows and irritations. Grandma always responded with advice, sympathy, love and humour.

All went well until the parents moved to Australia taking Peggy with them. There was no more meaningful communication between parents and child than there had ever been. The acute loss of the grandmother changed Peggy's character completely. The basic infantile rage which had always been there, but under cover, could no longer be hidden.

Peggy began to hate her parents, God and the world. In her early teens she developed suicidal tendencies. Her parents and those around them found her "a pain in the neck". No-one could understand what had happened to the friendly, docile little girl they had known. In their despair, Peggy's parents took her to a specially recommended doctor. He was an elderly man, a wise old soul. During a few consultations with the family, he recognised the picture and recommended a Rudolph Steiner school for the girl so that her character could be developed in another direction.

The parents were only too willing. During her years at the school, Peggy became happy, calm and outward-directed. She no longer felt that she was at fault in regard to her obnoxious behaviour or that she had been the cause of her parents' unhappiness.

The loving grandmother meanwhile died on the other side of the world and Peggy never saw her again. As a young adult, Peggy came into the presence of a sensitive one day, a medium. Her "dead" grandmother communicated, reminding Peggy of a few experiences she and the little one had shared years ago, and letting her know that she was with Peggy a great deal, helping and supporting her at every turn.

Peggy wholeheartedly accepted the communication and was very grateful for it. In her great love for Granny she did all she could to become more and more positive, knowing now that she was never alone. Granny guided her to follow through on her fine creative ability.

Peggy has become a successful fashion designer. In her spare time she explains to others just how the law of cause and effect operates. Two months before this writing, she met her affinity. The wedding will take place at Christmas-time. The two fine young people will walk hand in hand towards the same goal. They have both learned the lesson of giving and receiving true love from the point of self-respect and fulfilment in the world. Their future is bound to be a joyful one.

Chapter 10.4 - Poverty

Jack was over sixty when he came to consult us. The medium told him right away that he had been an unbonded baby, starved of love by both father and mother. He had no difficulty in realising this and in understanding that he had been looking for parental love from other people all his life. He had also been punishing those nearest to him as stand-ins for the parents, at whom he was basically very angry for letting him down early on when he was totally dependent on their love and encouragement for his development.

His father had not been a positive example for him to imitate safely. Young Jack realised soon enough that somehow he had to make his own way in life, despite his parents rather than with their moral support. His had been a drab and lonely childhood, with plenty of criticism and demands placed upon him. Jack decided to make his way in life by learning how to do business, after floundering a bit in the labour market as a very young man.

He got married in his twenties. Years later the marriage ended but Jack seemed quite indifferent to all that now.

The medium told him that she saw him being influenced primarily by two past incarnations so far in this life. One had been a very positive one as a North American Indian. He had totally fulfilled himself then in all aspects of living, acquiring great strength and stoicism as well as a basic sense of humour. These qualities had sustained him through his childhood and adulthood in this life, so that he did not come to any grievous harm despite the built-in deprivation and identity crisis.

However, he was much bothered and hampered by what he had brought along from his very last incarnation before the present one when he had been a priest in holy orders all his adult life. His own immortal self wanted to shed the characteristics and habits he had taken on then, and spread its wings in the present life, finally fulfilling its purpose by using its splendid talents of ancient days.

The conditioning for which he had opted in this monastic life had to be de-programmed by bringing its details fully into his present consciousness, so that he would no longer blindly repeat the old thought and behaviour pattern without knowing what he was doing, thus sabotaging his interests.

We started with the vow of poverty, explaining that this had not meant that he would be poverty-stricken in the ordinary sense, as the religious order was obliged to take care of his basic needs throughout his life, meaning he did not necessarily have to make a living. What it meant was, that from the time he took his final vows, he would no longer own any personal, private property or money any more. Everything would be "community property". If there were any financial gain from the work he did, it would go to the order, not to himself. The labourer was definitely not worthy of his hire.

The medium then saw him, in that life, promoted to serve in the Vatican itself because of his excellent business and organising abilities. There he had been active in creating wealth for the Vatican while still living the spartan life of a priest in holy orders.

At this point Jack burst out: "Oh, my God!" I worked for a multi-national company for thirty years. I made them millions of pounds every year, yet I was content with a salary of £30,000. I never even occurred to me that I should have a sizeable stake in those profits".

"The reason I wanted to come to see you is that when I retired a few years ago from the company, I was given the usual golden handshake. I invested it in a business of my own which lost money. I sold at a loss. Then I went into another business which is essentially a loser. Yet, when I worked for the big company I was much too shrewd to make such mistakes".

We pointed out to Jack that, deep in his psyche, he would have felt profoundly guilty about breaking the vow of poverty made in his last life. Unconsciously, he had been doing his best to get rid of all his personal, private property which caused him so much discomfort.

Now, knowing what was going on, he could stop sabotaging his success, and demonstrate to the world what he could do when he was following through on his inspiration. His self-sabotage had blocked his intuition at every turn.

Jack was so impressed with what had already come to light in his session with us, and so eager to set things right in his life that we all agreed to stop right there and let him get on with it. Other matters could be sorted out at a later date if he so desired. After all, his business situation was an emergency. He ran to catch the next train back to salvage what was left.

Chapter 10.5 - The Aztec Princess

Myra is a professional woman in her fifties. Her parents had been in harmony with one another both before and for years after Myra's birth. The mother was undemonstrative as she herself had been raised that way. Little Myra therefore had some deep-seated anger in her, but felt more secure than most children until she was nearly five years old.

The grown-up Myra, already a grandparent, came to see us because of a very disagreeable symptom which had plagued her so many times in her life that she could not remember all the incidences. She would suddenly develop an uncontrollable watery diarrhoea, sometimes with, more often without, accompanying vomiting. Between these episodes she was perfectly alright, often for months or even a year or more.

The official diagnosis had always been "a stomach bug" or "intestinal 'flu" and an especial susceptibility to this kind of thing. Over the years Myra had recognised a pattern in her symptomatology that did not at all agree with this kind of diagnosis. She had noticed that there was a strong connection with journeys by car or by train, never by air. The association with travel made the symptoms particularly embarrassing, and Myra had learned to have medication containing a small amount of opium in her handbag at such times. The opium, taken regularly from the first inkling of a loose stool, would slow the hyperactive intestinal activity down to a tolerable level, but Myra objected to the slight impairment of her mental acuity by the medication. She never drank alcoholic beverages and enjoyed being wide awake and aware at all times in her life.

The medium was given the cause of Myra's repetitive symptom of diarrhoea in a long past life-time in which Myra, as the beautiful young daughter of an Aztec Indian king, had been selected to be ritually sacrificed to the Aztec deity. The girl confronted her father with the idea that, if he loved her as she thought he did, he would save her from this fate. The king was more concerned with upholding the old custom than with his daughter's wish. Feeling utterly let down by her father whom she had trusted, the girl, not at all impressed by the "honour" bestowed upon her, escaped from the capital to an outlying area where she was kindly taken in by a woman of the people.

It must be interjected here that, as the medium was inspired with salient features of this life-time, Myra rapidly had recollections of it herself out of her deep unconscious memory. Therefore, many details became available especially as Myra herself recognised several souls in the long past life as prior incarnations of persons she knew in the present one. Now to go on with the story:

The Aztec princess knew that her escape from being made a human sacrifice was itself a crime punishable by death. Yet she felt relatively safe in the simple abode of the woman. Meanwhile, back home, a reward was offered for anyone who would find and return the fugitive to the capital. A minor functionary coveted this reward. He knew of his psychic ability and used it to divine the princess's hiding place. With a few soldiers he went and collected her and the woman who had tried to save her from her fate. The two were bound and roughly transported back to the royal enclave. There they were placed on adjacent slabs in a dark chamber to be executed by having their throats cut.

Myra remembered the first time she had the severe diarrhoea and vomiting when she was nearly five years old. She was ill for a number of days then, unable to do anything. The episode had been preceded by a move from the part of the country where Myra had been born, a sunny part with friendly neighbours, to the city where her parents' relatives lived. There the sky was overcast and her grandmother's flat dark and dreary, actually because it looked out on a park whose tall trees shaded the windows in the summer. The journey itself had been made in an old railway carriage with hard wooden seats and two strange men in the same compartment. Myra's father had gone ahead earlier, so that she was travelling only with her mother. The journey lasted through the night.

Looking back, Myra could easily see that the involuntary, somewhat primitive journey from a home and friends she had enjoyed to a "dark" place and people with whom she felt nothing in common cued her right into the as yet unresolved total terror and feeling of betrayal of the transportation to doom and destruction in the Aztec experience. The symptoms were those of abject fear and revulsion. The little girl in the twentieth century recovered, of course, but as a child was never again as happy as she had been in the land of her birth.

It is now quite a number of years since Myra was helped to become conscious of the cause of her symptoms. She had made many more journeys overland without any difficulty whatsoever. However, she came back to us later because of another symptom which she had first had at the age of thirteen. It had also recurred many times. What characterised it was an acute and sudden pain in the heart region, accompanied by a feeling of not being able to inhale properly resulting in small gasps for air. Any attempt to breathe more deeply would intensify the pain quite intolerably. The episode would invariably last only a number of minutes, gradually abating. It might, however, recur several times a day for a few days.

Despite the concern of those around her when she was briefly afflicted in this way, Myra had never been afraid that there might be any heart condition. She had been told that such pain was easily produced by an intercostal (between the ribs) muscle spasm. The symptom had recurred for the first time in a number of years when she came back to see us. She had spent a rainy, cold summer in a small hotel. The cold weather had robbed her of the pleasure of part of her time off. Myra's absolutely solid conviction that the pain, though perceived in the heart region, had nothing at all to do with the heart was quite remarkable in a lady of middle age.

The medium was promptly shown the origin of the pain. She saw Myra once more as the Aztec princess lying on the slab, ready to be executed in the dim chamber used for this purpose. Her father, the king, came in. He was holding a knife-like instrument. The cutting of the throat was going to be a rather prolonged, gruesome affair with the primitive equipment available. The father had come to spare his daughter this final ordeal by stabbing her through the heart quickly in advance. He pierced her chest with a powerful stroke.

At this moment of the medium's transmission, Myra's own memory rose as she exclaimed: "Oh, my God! He couldn't even do that right! He just missed my heart. My lungs filled with blood. The pain was horrendous. I gasped for air, the movement increasing the pain still more. I just remember the horror of a few short gasps then nothing more."

Myra realised that the dank, cold, dreary weather conditions which restrained her holiday freedom and possibly a disappointment about the loyalty of a colleague shortly before had cued her into the as yet unresolved remnant of the Aztec experience. She did not think she would ever feel her stabbing pain in the "heart" again now. As of this writing she has not had it.

One other thing which impressed Myra was that, in recognising the souls who had been her father and her captor in the Aztec life in their present-day incarnations, she was aware how little they had actually learned since that time about becoming or being positive people. They were still about learning some of the same lessons as before, and Myra had given each of them another opportunity to learn this time around. It was still too soon to see whether they would take it or not, but the likelihood seemed small.

Myra's spirit had given these opportunities long before the Myra personality knew anything about the distant past. Her generous, loving permanent Self had planned the life that way. Its own interests had also been intertwined with this generosity. Myra had had to learn to detach herself from people who were not ready to change, thus going precisely nowhere. For Myra it had been a hard learning to stop pouring her own energy into souls who would not or could not yet make and sustain their own effort to progress. Trying to force their progress had been a form of manipulation, an interference with natural law.

Chapter 11

Negativity

Basically, negativity is the denial of self, the God-self which is the cause of every incarnation. How does this denial come into being?

For the answer to this question we have to look once again to the earliest part of a human existence, the pre-natal and post-natal time. When, instead of being joyfully and warmly welcomed, the newcomer is either isolated or rejected. Fear develops, followed by anger as the only available survival mechanism. The response to fear in man and beast alike is fight or flight. As the basic emotions are carried along in the growing and grown human being, the result will be a personality which gets defensive at every turn, as soon as anything or anybody - a circumstance, a word, a look - cues the subconscious child into its early life experience. In this vulnerable state the individual will defend himself not only against other people but also against the God-self, which the inner child early began to misidentify with its depriving, rejecting or threatening elders.

There is also the feeling that aggression is the best defence. So, when the anger predominates, attack is inevitable. This can take a number of forms, depending on the basic constitution of a person as well as examples seen in parent figures and treatment received from them. In some relatively fiery individuals the anger will build up to an intolerable point and suddenly be released in a temper tantrum, usually leaving others in the environment shattered. Less fiery adults may evidence a "slow toil", simmering away, exuding sharpness, quarrelling, cynicism, nastiness and offensiveness of every description. Here again, the true self is held at bay and itself attacked by the personality which confuses it with the natural parents of the inner little one.

Fear and rage tend to lead to rebellion which originally was simply a show of strength, often put down and maligned by those in charge of the child. The rebellion needs to seek an outlet which it can find in sundry people, institutions or conditions onto whom or which the sufferer projects the original situation.

Another favourite target for the anger and the rebellion is the sufferer's own body and health. Especially when in childhood there were heavy penalties for any open expression of these emotions, the physical self as well as the soul is attacked. The result is assorted abuse of the body, such as subjecting it to inadequate diets, poisons, drugs or violent stress and strain. Another mode is the development of neurotic symptoms or disease. These, then, are also indicators of deep-rooted guilt feelings due to earlier accusations and condemnations, often in response to adverse criticism and hard or harsh discipline. Guilt feelings invariably and quickly lead to self-punishment. This way not only the personality but also its loving owner, the spirit, is punished. The latter then cannot function as it needs to do through a channel which is busy flagellating and sabotaging itself at every turn.

The anger is not always just from the pre-natal period or childhood. Very often it has also been brought along from the incarnation just left behind or sometimes from an even earlier one. Then the angering circumstances early on in the present life serve to bring the old rage to the surface so that it can hopefully be dealt with and resolved at some time during the life rather than be carried along any further.

As there is nothing but thought (consciousness) in all the universe, it cannot be surprising that all this fear, anger, rebellion and ill-feeling about self and the world hangs around planet Earth like smog in the atmosphere of a modern city. Like attracts like. Therefore, when an individual, a group or a nation is in a state of infantile misery, this is automatically reinforced from the communal pool of similar emotions. Many people, even whole peoples, are then trapped in this morass, this vicious circle.

One can also put it this way: The general pool of negativity will seek to penetrate any Achilles heel offered by an individual to make things worse and keep the individual from learning to love self and fulfilling self. There is no doubt that negativity is a strong force; but love is stronger.

Let us not forget that anger is the force provided by nature as the one and only mechanism for surviving killer fear. Man has pronounced it evil. This is a deception which has caused guilt, still more fear and yet more anger and rebellion. By now all humanity is suffering from a war against the Higher Self, the only real self. It is continuously preoccupied with this form of despair and denies itself insight into the manipulations of the mortal personality - until the cycle has run its course. This is like one great tantrum which finally ends in peace.

The infantile state in adults has a number of other characteristics, again depending on the early environment and the factors brought along from other lifetimes and expressing as character.

If the child has been deprived of love or been rejected, it may react by continuing the pattern in self-deprivation of rejection of self. On the other hand, its unfilled need for love combined with anger and rebellion may make it greedy later. Here we find the people for whom the acquisition of money or goods becomes the be-all and end-all of their existence. Some of these will hoard what they gain or collect obsessively; others will destroy anyone or anything getting in the way of their fruitless pursuit which can never bring them what they truly want - love and peace. As the small child is by definition weak and powerless, such people are often equally greedy for power, power at all costs, in the subconscious attempt to counteract their basic lack of self-esteem and their deeply-felt vulnerability.

In any case these states will be reinforced from the surrounding pool of negativity. Often such people also attract others of their own kind, either as "partners in crime" or as adversaries, or both.

Looked at from this angle, it is easy to see how many appalling conditions on this planet have come about, but also that, once all is out in the open, resolution will be found.

Chapter 11.2 - Intellect

There has occurred in human civilisation an over-development of the intellect. It is a major component of the earthly personality. Along with the emotions it is conditioned early in life and onward. In fact, the emotions and the intellect become functionally intertwined, each stimulating the other to mischief.

We like to compare the intellect with a computer. It works just fine and is very useful indeed when it has been soundly programmed and a skilled operator is handling it. Good programming would arise from positive conditioning early in life resulting in solid self-respect and plenty of natural pride: a fine self-image. This would automatically ensure that the only possible skilled operator, the spirit, would direct and use the intellect to capacity with perfect judgement and clarity of purpose. This operator is superbly intelligent and knowledgeable and does not make mistakes. All is well and enjoyable.

If, however, the early conditioning caused basic defects like lack of self-esteem, the spirit is prevented from calmly running the machine. The intellect runs amok, driven by very personal emotional concerns of an essentially infantile nature. Instead of adult actions, there are mainly reactions, chains of them, each feeding into the next. There is entirely unproductive or counter-productive repetitive thinking, round and round, over and over the same old territory. This deadly monotony is a bore to the personality as well as to the spirit. If any of it is verbally expressed, it makes a similar impression on the listener. This, indeed, is negativity in another form. It can hardly take place when no words are permitted to form by a determined outer consciousness. The words used in circular "word thinking", supplied by one's own language memory bank, are the favourite ammunition used by negativity against one's own self to prevent one from succeeding in any forward-looking enterprise.

One need not put up with this nasty trick. One can practice being aware and awake and active in daily life, not permitting undesirable phrases, sentences, paragraphs or whole pages of words to run through one's head. Repeated practice for a week in the spirit of gamesmanship, with negativity as one's opponent, brings considerable blessed relief.

We have often said that circular or discursive word thinking is used as a barrage against the spirit self which cannot "get a word in edgewise" under such conditions. This leaves the personality feeling miserable and unattended, a state desired by negativity as an opening for the production of further shambles.

Man is a habit-forming creature. But his habits need not be permanent by any means. If he diligently practices a new habit for a very short time, it will promptly replace the accustomed one of which he desires to rid himself. This is particularly easy if he has been helped to clear up the faulty early conditioning which might otherwise still drive him to sabotage his own success.

Chapter 11.3 - Aches and Pains case history

Eric, a computer specialist, was in his late thirties when he came to see us. He thought we might be able to help him with his assorted physical symptoms, mainly neck and back pain. He claimed these nagging aches and pains which no-one had been able to alleviate kept him from relaxing and enjoying himself.

Within minutes we perceived that his outlook on life was miserable. He could not see any sense in living, yet he was afraid of dying. He looked at life as a great punishment, insisting that suffering was the price one had to pay for being bad. He was an utter pessimist and obviously spent time trying to drag others down with him into his sullen denial of everything that was worthwhile.

He could not see the beauty of nature. It disturbed him to be in happy surroundings, to see others enjoying themselves. He cared nothing for others except that they be an audience for him. Even animals meant nothing to him. From morning to night he was totally self-centred and full of self-pity. He talked about himself continuously to those around him and became known as "Misery Eric".

Apparent to everyone was his phenomenal anger. He had a viper's tongue and woe betide anyone who was willing to listen to his wailing. His negative thought force was so strong that before long, he would pull the listener down to his own level of misery, leaving him or her feeling unhappy too. His insistent talk had a hypnotic quality with which he would instill his own state into the consciousness of the other person, while vilifying everything and everybody.

He came to us as a last resort, saying: "I can't stand myself. I know I'm awful. I can't find any relief". We found the cause of his state mainly in his pre-natal and post-natal experience. He was the second child of a woman who did not like men and already had one son. She was not happy about being pregnant and wished that this child at least should be a daughter. Needless to say, the incoming soul knew it was in a male body and therefore felt all wrong, completely rejected. The mother was a complaining, long-suffering sort herself. As if all that were not enough, when Eric was a week old his twenty-two months older brother came down with paralytic polio, henceforth losing the use of both his legs and having to be put back into a pram until he was old enough to have surgery, full braces and crutches. The mother's wailing can be imagined.

Obviously the baby could not rationally comprehend what was going on and literally "imbibed" the mother's state with her milk. Already feeling unwanted and wrong from this pre-natal experience, he was automatically certain that he himself was the cause of all mother's sorrowfulness and profound self-pity.

The father was a kind and cheerful man but too passive for his wife. He could not handle her negativity. Besides, he had to work for a living and help look after the paralysed boy in his spare time. The baby had little close contact with his father for some time.

Eric could see the implications of his early history to the way he felt about himself and the world. Again and again, he would relax a few moments and let go of his misery. We hoped that any moment he would acquire a permanent insight and a sense of humour about himself. It was a vain hope. However many angles of approach we tried, success was only momentary. Invariably Eric fell back into his accustomed morbidity. Finally he demanded that we make his entire effort for him. Failing that, he became argumentative and we had to terminate the session.

Through a common acquaintance we were informed of further developments in Eric's life. Though he had not basically altered, he got married. Eventually there were two children and one on the way. The wife always had a difficult time with her husband, as can be imagined. During her third pregnancy Eric one day informed her that he simply had to go to India to find himself a guru. He left and that was the last anyone has seen or heard of him. His now aged father is helping his daughter-in-law and the children as best he can.

Chapter 11.4 - Cancer case history

Ellen remembered how she felt when she was born: "Oh, my God, here I am and nobody wants me. I am cold". In fact, Ellen has felt cold ever since, wearing extra clothing most of the time. Everyone knows that warmth is perceived as a symbol for love. We speak of a warm heart. The absence of love is often perceived as coldness, like feeling out in the cold.

Before marriage, Ellen's mother had been a trained nanny. She raised her daughter "strictly by the book and the clock". Having been a rejected child herself, the mother could not enjoy her pregnancy or establish any meaningful communication with her child before or after birth. Ellen, who was the pregnancy, depended on a free and natural flow of love to and from her parent. She was bound to feel "out in the cold" and terribly afraid in her unnatural isolation. Intense fear prevents the firm uniting of body and soul at the proper time and rate and is, therefore, life-threatening. The little one's only defence is the development of intense anger which takes its energy from the fear, thus reducing the latter to a tolerable level. The anger, better termed infantile rage, is thus a valuable survival technique. Without it, there would have had to be a miscarriage or an early infant death.

Ellen remembers her parents' marriage as joyless, without even a pretence of mutual affection. When she was three or four years old, her father "lost everything", so that the family had to live in financially reduced circumstances. In Ellen's words, she remembers "being thrashed continuously, both at home and at school". At home she was beaten with a three-pronged whip until she was fourteen years old. She says that the idea of severe physical discipline is deeply rooted in the character of the population in the country where she grew up.

At twenty-one, Ellen married a scientist working for a large multi-national corporation. Genuine love was something Ellen had obviously never experienced. The marriage looked to her like a good way to get away from home. In line with the husband's work, the couple were moved from country to country for many years. They had six children by and by.

When Ellen first came to us for help, she had been married for thirty-five years. Her youngest child was twenty-two and working. Until the departure of the youngest, she had seen herself as very restricted in the family and felt that only now were things beginning to open out for her. She described her husband as extremely conventional, adding that he had been persecuting her all her life because of her spiritual interests. According to Ellen he hates women and had stopped having marital relations with her some years before. She added: "I find him immensely aggravating every day of my life".

In the Far East, Ellen had learned some techniques of traditional medical and meditation practices. She became a meditation teacher after returning to Britain. For many years she has been an active member of a quasi-religious group which brainwashed her into a set of strict rules and dogmas. Having taken this indoctrination on board, she was promoted to a minor leading and teaching role in the organisation. Part of the dogma is making the candidate feel guilty about leaving the organisation, and prohibiting the joining of any other religious group. It is a type of loyalty oath based on fear.

Physically Ellen had acute glaucoma in both eyes fifteen years ago, and now has the chronic variety, treated by drugs. She also complained of chronic "constriction problems in the stomach". She looked very thin and pale, almost translucent. Questions about her diet revealed that she was basically a vegetarian, almost a vegan, and on a low salt intake, all by her own prescription. She gave a history of repeated episodes of iron-deficiency anaemia. She had been drinking coffee several times daily and wine with her evening meals.

We gently explained to her that she had been able to survive the deprivation and fear of her pre-natal and post-natal period by means of the intense anger which had then remained with her all her life. As usual, such anger results in rebellion which, in her case, was later very much turned against herself. Her self-depriving and self-destructive activities had been learned very early and thoroughly from her environment.

She was counselled in detail, first of all to revise her diet to support rather than deprive her body in its functioning, and to stop attacking it with nutritional poisons. We pointed out to her that there were very concrete dangers to her health in her accustomed state of being. Born angry, she was now furious about the past as well as deeply resenting her present situation, especially her husband. Having had no positive role models in her parents, her life-long identity crisis predisposed her to seek a bogus identity in her extreme religious pursuits within an organisation as joyless as her parents' marriage. She had remained in her own marriage despite the fact that she loathed her husband. Her early and adult environments had caused her to sink deeper and deeper into negativity.

The medium pointed out that in a previous life Ellen had been a witch and learned the misuse of the power of thought. Ellen had no trouble accepting this information. She had herself wondered about it already. She had a habit of wallowing in always seeing the worst about people and events, pathologically latching on to prophecies of doom and destruction. Morbid thoughts of one or another sort persistently occupied her waking consciousness and her talk. Her remarkable psychic gifts were put at the service of negativity while she deluded herself into thinking she was a "spiritual" person. Her habits of negative thinking and feeling were the perfect recipe for very severe illness if not altered in good time.

Ellen promised to eat more sensibly. She did not want to separate from her husband or to free herself up from the brainwashing organisation. The minor post she occupied in it flattered her.

Two years after the first session Ellen came to see us again, saying that for the last three weeks she had been suffering from the worst cold she had ever had, feeling very ill with it.

Asked what had happened in her life, she said that two weeks before the onset of symptoms, her husband had informed her that he had been having an affair with another woman for some time already, and that he was planning to live with the lady after his forthcoming retirement. Ellen, though noticing a great relief in herself, at the same time felt severely betrayed.

We pointed out to her that now was a great time for her to let her positive, innermost self demonstrate its honesty and generosity; to show everybody who and what she really was underneath her thick veneer of acquired negativity. Here was a splendid opportunity for her to turn around completely, to make a new and independent life for herself right now and enable her husband to be equally free and without guilt.

Meanwhile, Ellen generally looked much better, having fed herself more sensibly after seeing us two years before.

She felt there was much common sense in our ideas and she would give the matter some serious thought.

Although we never again saw Ellen professionally, she stayed in touch and we met her with fair frequency. She did find herself a new place to live, and started to do more of her own work. Her husband helped her where he could, materially, to make her own way. Though she was glad to live on her own, there remained a great resentment. Her tie-in with the organisation continued unabated. Ellen was masterly at deluding herself as to the true nature of her feelings and the real motives for her actions. Rationalisation had always been easy for her. Her great talents, despite much encouragement from us and others, were still used to mix obvious truths with less obvious falsehoods, a favourite ploy of negativity to get the recipient to swallow the pill. Destructive criticism still remained a frequent activity.

Another two years had passed when we had a distress call from Ellen. As her "stomach constrictions" had never ceased, she had once again sought medical help. No physical cause had ever been found for this symptom which is quite a common expression of emotional imbalance. None was found this time either, but a much more generalised examination led to the discovery of a cancerous growth which had not yet given rise to any symptoms at all. We and others gave Ellen every conceivable positive support to help her through a prolonged and very difficult period of disagreeable preliminary assessments in hospital, very major and successful surgery following, and a necessarily lengthy period of adjustment afterwards.

The surgeon, who knew Ellen's life situation, of his own accord told her that the real cause of her tumour had to be her profound resentment against her husband. Ellen told us herself that she had been quite unaware that this emotion was still there, but could see it when the surgeon pointed it out. She now set about actively to let go of the resentment. Aware that she could easily do herself further serious harm with her negativity, she became quite a different person, fun to be with. She had an intelligent and delightful sense of humour, was full of amusing anecdotes and interesting bits of knowledge from her vast store of experience in many countries.

Alas, when everyone was beginning to believe that she had really turned the corner, Ellen did not sustain her effort in the direction of positivity. The honeymoon was over. She fell right back into her old pattern of negativity, trying to manipulate other people, criticising, undermining and mixing truth with falsehood. She has missed three great opportunities to come into her own, and she may not have a fourth one in this life.

Chapter 12

Depression

The package of infantile despair, as I call it, consists of:

a)   Feeling unbonded, i.e. unloved, unwelcomed and often actually rejected, unwanted, even a calamity.

b)   Fear, even terror, resulting from a parent's wish or attempt to abort.

c)   Anger, called infantile rage, as the only survival mechanism in the face of killer fear ("I'm frightened to death").

d)   Rebellion, a simple show of strength in the young, not at all appreciated by the responsible adults.

The non-bonding and/or rejecting parent figures also set negative examples upon which the young cannot safely mould themselves.

An identity crisis is the result. The children grow up not knowing who or what they really are. They are walking on ice, slithering hither and yon, feeling insecure, needy, unloved and unlovable. The divinity which has fashioned them, their own immortal spirit, is not only not recognised by them under these circumstances, but actually fought off. It is perceived to be as the parents were, untrustworthy.

These matters are not intellectual processes. They happen on the level of repressed memories, the emotions, the feelings. The subconscious is in charge as the individual matures physically. It is primitive, not rational. It was never meant to be the leader. It needs to be under the control of the loving spirit just like a car has to be steered by the driver.

This kind of problem is not new, of course. It has been propagated by whole cultures on this earth for countless generations. Therefore, many souls incarnating are still afflicted by the consequences of previous life-times spent under its shadow. They bring some of their fear, their anger, their willfulness and stubbornness with them. These traits are then caused to surface in the young by the lack of love, support and encouragement from equally afflicted parents.

The spirit, being divine, is creative. Man's soul or spirit is part of the totality, of the Creator. It is, therefore, in his very nature to create. A child taken to a sandy beach will start constructing sandcastles, canals, whole towns, or a cake. Given crayons and paper, it will draw; given vehicles it will make them run and perform work. A youngster tries out to see what can be done with available materials, even if there is nothing but sticks and pebbles, and invariably enjoys using the imagination.

Each human being has urges to make things, organise things, set something up, construct something, tangible or intangible. However much or little creativity there is in a person it must be used. Of course, some people have more talent than others, but none are without. If creativity is denied its expression, if it is blocked by "I cannot", "I must not", "I may not", or "I shall not", the soul itself is thwarted and feels shackled or trapped. Under these circumstances the personality, the temporary self, cannot feel happy. The anger and spite increase. In fact, the personality is distressed. This state is then referred to as depression.

If a man does not know what is niggling him, he makes up something which justifies his being angry. He can always find some circumstance or person in his environment to blame. At the same time he seeds compassion from others. To get his way he tries to make himself interesting. There is much showing off then in a variety of ways to draw attention or to get pity and compassion focussed on him. This attention raises the self-image a little; but the comfort is short-lived. The great anger and frustration about not having been able to create to capacity remains.

As a personality continues to reject or suppress its innate creativity, a state of utter boredom develops, self-created through apathy or stupidity. Finally, depression becomes a habit. As anyone who has been depressed or lived with a person subject to depression knows, some of the anger tends to be ventilated in that state, often with explosive suddenness, leading to a temporary improvement.

A permanent cure is only obtained through the freeing up of the sufferer's creativity into action. This brings joy and a deep satisfaction.

Depression is a very common condition indeed in civilisations where a multitude of rusty old customs and habits are proof of an abysmal ignorance of what life is really all about. These neurotic or even psychotic cultural patterns try to subdue, even to kill off, the very essence of what it means to be a human being, free and creative. Something has to be done about this horrendous state of affairs.

Creativity is of the essence for man. Its prime importance has not been sufficiently recognised.

It can be expressed in every aspect of life, in thought, word and deed, in little things as well as in great ones. This is a true need of man's nature, be he young or old. There is nothing infantile about it. Creation brings joyfulness in its wake, as it is joy in action.

When parents are aware that they are manufacturing and nurturing a body for an incoming soul, they will feel a great satisfaction in this most creative task that human beings can undertake, namely responsible and loving parenting. It prepares another generation for freely creative expression from the start! Such parenthood has to become a chain reaction which eliminates what is called "depression" at the source.

Children, adolescents and young adults need to be guided, supported, encouraged and trained to use all the creative drive they have. They must be made aware of its desirability and its great importance to themselves and to society. Appreciation for their originality, their constructive ideas and accomplishments goes a long way toward furthering a truly adult and responsible generation. It should be remembered that the need to create is not sex-linked. Boys and girls are equally creative. Only the body is of one or the other sex. The soul or spirit is of the Divine. Here now are a few clinical examples of active interference with a child's creative potential:

Little Annie's mother had been a fine professional soprano before she was married. From an early age, Annie was aware that the pregnancy and her birth had "ruined her mother's voice". In her teens Annie was discovered to be at least as good a soprano as her mother had been. She was sent to a well-known singing teacher who supposedly "ruined" her voice for ever after. No-one realised that Annie was actually punishing herself for having supposedly spoilt her mother's singing.

At the same time, Annie did not want to give her mother an opportunity for a vicarious satisfaction, not after all those years of undermining. These motives remained unconscious until thirty more years had passed and it was much too late for Annie's voice to be developed. However, she did discover herself to be an excellent writer and now writes for publication.

Then there was little Billy. His father was very gifted in art and sculpture. However, he was very self-centred at home. He did not bother with his son, and had no real interest in or patience with him, leaving the raising and training to the mother and other relatives. The boy showed promise early on along the father's line of talents. However, long before kindergarten age, he no longer wanted to do anything with art materials. When strongly encouraged to try, he produced primitive and repetitive things, becoming more and more angry while doing them. Even in adult life, Bill could not control the situation, though his choice of colours and furnishings in the home as well as his clothing showed unmistakably artistic talent.

He was already a grandfather when we were able to make it clear to him that he had felt utterly rejected by his father and correspondingly angry at him, therefore rebelling against that within himself which was like his father.

Bill saw the funny side of the rebellious little boy in his subconscious. He promptly enrolled in adult education art classes. Having taken the reins off his own talent, he became a capable instructor himself in time, enjoying every minute. He still laughs about his own story.

Chapter 12.2 - A Sore Toe case history

Edward was the child of aristocratic parents. From birth he was cared for by nannies, being presented to his parents at specified times, all dressed up for the visit. At other times, one or the other of his parents would visit the nursery to see that the children were well cared for, and to become a little better acquainted with them. This was the way father and mother had been brought up themselves. The pattern was the "done thing", blindly repeated for another generation.

Edward's memories of his early years were scant and bland, his parents shadowy figures in the background. At seven years of age he was sent to an upper class boarding school. He remembers being very unhappy there for some time. Bullied by older boys, he was unable to defend himself and tended to withdraw into a corner. He was subjected to the usual pranks, like having a brush placed under his sheet and having one or another of his belongings hidden away. At times he would be given a false message by the boys. Particularly poignant among these was the seriously communicated bogus news that his father had died. The practical jokes were without end. Even though the little boys became older boys, the tantalising continued in one way or another. It was tradition. Discipline was of the usual strict variety and all the boys were trained into the acceptable "stiff upper lip" mentality. This meant that they were to hide their true feelings as much as they could and must never give way to strong emotions, not even admit them to themselves. Free expression was not the done thing.

Meanwhile, Edward's parents travelled many years abroad. His school holidays were spent with relatives or in the company of strangers as arranged for him. He was definitely the poor child of rich parents.

Never having been a good student, he could not finish his A levels, and left school without qualifications and with no idea of what to do with his life.

He was not practical with his hands. A very sensitive person, he liked music and poetry. He loved animals and adored walking alone over downs and fields, especially in Scotland and Wales, musing as he walked. For years he had a repetitive dream in which he saw himself standing on a raised platform speaking to an assembly of people with his arms outstretched, giving them a kind of blessing.

In his late teens, Edward got mixed up with a religious sect which demanded total sacrifice and surrender to "God". It forbade any further contact with parents, relatives or friends. Instead, there was to be absolute obedience to those at the head of the organisation who ran it. After a couple of years Edward had grown up enough to see through the motives of the founder of the sect. Disillusioned, he managed to get out.

Edward's health troubles began with excruciating pain in a big toe. It became swollen. He had great difficulty walking on it or wearing proper shoes. No immediate cause for the trouble was found, and a walking stick was suggested. Limping along, Edward made the acquaintance of a friendly old man who told him that he was a spiritual healer. In his misery, Edward eagerly accepted his services. The very next morning the swelling was gone. There was only a slight redness and residual soreness left.

When Edward first put on a decent pair of shoes again, he bent down to tie his laces and found that he could not straighten up because of a very severe pain in his back. He had lumbago. There was no choice but to spend days in bed, incapacitated. The immobility was terribly boring. Then, as suddenly as it had appeared, the pain was gone again.

For a whole week Edward was well. Then he had a blinding headache along with nausea. He felt very ill indeed. A doctor came and examined him. The diagnosis was migraine. Tablets relieved the symptoms to some extent, so that Edward could at least function. The migraine returned again at irregular intervals.

Gradually Edward became more and more unsure of himself. The consecutive symptomatology plagued him. He developed pains in his heart region and shortness of breath while walking, yet nothing could be found wrong with his heart. Then a chronic form of hayfever was added to his miseries. As soon as one of the older symptoms cleared up, it was replaced by another.

Friends told Edward that he was a hypochondriac. In his despair he went to see a specialist in Internal Medicine who suggested a psychiatrist. The latter told Edward to come for a therapy hour twice a week for six months and then they would take stock and see how to go on from there. Edward dutifully went for his sessions, though all this was financially quite hard for him. After three months he felt no better and became restless. One weekend he went to a local health exhibition. There he talked with a lady who is an aromatherapist. She told him about our work. He then acquired some literature about us and it made sense to him.

As he had run out of money by this time, he borrowed some to come to see us. Quickly and easily we could show him that in his whole life he had never experienced any love at all. His parents, unbonded themselves, could not bond with their children. Edward's earliest feelings were of loneliness and isolation and the fear generated by these unnatural conditions. To continue on earth he had had to develop and sustain abiding anger, which he had later turned upon himself. Never having been enjoyed or appreciated, he could not enjoy or appreciate himself, nor did he feel entitled to a joyful existence. Only animals had given him their simple, uncomplicated love and he could love them in return.

The way he was raised he had no positive adult role models after which to fashion himself, so that he grew up quite at sea about his own identity. What he saw and experienced in his many years at boarding school was foreign to his deeply sensitive nature. The abuse there undermined him even more.

His inner child's desperate need for loving parents made him easy prey for the sect which caught him for two years of his young adulthood. The maturity of his innermost eternal self was shown by the fact that he saw through the motives of the organisation and distanced himself from it despite the brainwashing he had already been given. Yet then he found himself once more on his own, disappointed again by people whom he had trusted in his despair. He also blamed himself for having fallen for their tricks and for being an underachiever in life, not knowing where to turn.

The anger at himself was the cause of the symptoms he had developed. Clearly, they were subconsciously designed to rob him of the one activity he was really able to enjoy, his long walks through the hills and fields.

Whenever there are guilt feelings of any kind, and they are never reasonable, self-punishment does not lag far behind. None of this sequence need be fully conscious; but the end result are pain, discomfort or despair certainly is. The feelings of deprivation, fear, anger and rebellion and their concomitant identity crisis together make up the infantile package commonly referred to as depression. They may surface at any time in adult life. Some experience which is strongly reminiscent of the original one in infancy will light the fuse, causing the more or less dormant bomb to explode. Another sign of the maturity of Edward's soul was the fact that his "bomb" smouldered rather than exploded, meaning that he had not become mentally ill, just neurotic. At no time had he lost his hold on reality.

Edward's repetitive "dream" of long standing was not really a dream but a memory of another life-time, one lived in India. He had become a beloved teacher of the masses there, one who was whole and wholesome in himself, fulfilled and joyful in his life. He had been able to teach by his example of positivity. The unconscious recollection of this state of wholeness had sustained him and given him the strength in the present life to come through as he had despite the circumstances. Somewhere he had always known that there was light at the end of the tunnel, that he could be whole again.

The life in India was some time ago. In his last incarnation, Edward had made some mistakes. Raised harshly in a fundamentalist Christian belief, he had become a missionary. Sent to convert a primitive but natural people, he had done his best to teach them all about sin, guilt and punishment, foisting his own inculcated ideas on their previously unselfconscious, relaxed state of being. He had regarded these people as heathens as he had been taught.

For the present incarnation as Edward, he had again chosen a loveless, harsh childhood and adolescent environment in the knowledge that he could overcome the deficit. Again sucked into a dogmatic belief system, he had freed himself from it, not repeating his past error.

It now remained for Edward to get to know his true Self, the permanent one; to learn to love it and to accept its love and wisdom. Then he would be in the light at the end of his tunnel and able to teach again through his own wholeness, though in a totally modern setting.

Edward has come to see us altogether three times over a period of two years. He has taken on a position in management on his father's estate where he is engaged in promoting organic farming, a goal close to his heart. He had already known quite a bit about the subject and is making it a study in depth with real enthusiasm. His father seems relieved and happy that one of his sons is actively engaged in this field. In fact, the two men, formerly almost strangers, have become friends, learning from each other.

Edward is now aware that he has always had psychic gifts; that he is very much a sensitive and as an "old" soul was bound to feel lonely in any setting where there was no-one on his own level of spiritual maturity, no-one with whom he could communicate in a meaningful way. As he has always loved music and poetry, he is now learning to play the flute, to read music and also to do some creative writing of his own in his spare time.

With all these efforts at self-expression his self-esteem and enjoyment level are constantly rising. His habit of self-criticism has been receding more and more, and his psychosomatic symptoms along with it. We have reminded him that "Rome wasn't built in a day", that being impatient with himself is just another way of being intolerant with self, a further attack on his own soul. He is still young and it does not matter at all that the habits of another life-time take a while to unload. In fact, every time he slips, he gets another impetus to move forward as these slips are very uncomfortable. After more years filled with life experience, Edward will again be teaching through his new-found wholeness and its accompanying success in his material life. The particular form which his teaching will take will be up to his wise eternal Self. Right now he already serves as a shining example of relentless progression to his own environment. He is a joy for all who know him.

Chapter 12.3 - Escaping Despair

Walter came on time for his appointment in the afternoon. We started to work with him. After twenty minutes, it was painfully obvious to both of us that we were not getting anywhere at all. Walter was very willing and very cooperative, but that did not do any good. He was not able to comprehend anything worthwhile.

We felt as if we were trying to reach Walter through a padded wall around his consciousness. Having had this kind of experience before, one of us asked him when he had last had an alcoholic beverage to drink. The previous evening he had had several glasses of beer.

We asked him whether he was feeling "all there", and he wasn't, really. Then we explained that, although his bloodstream would no longer contain alcohol so many hours later, his brain would not have recovered yet. We carefully and slowly told him that the cell-membrane of brain cells is made of an extremely thin layer of lipid, a waxy substance; that, as alcohol is a fat-solvent, it attacks this membrane, even making holes in it which are visible under an electron microscope. We pointed out that brain cells in such a condition are not functioning as they should, and require from two to seven days to heal if not attacked again in the meantime.

Walter had to accept that to continue the session with us would be a waste of our energy and his money. We would rather take the afternoon off. He had come a long way but could see the simple logic of the situation. In fact, he was very impressed by being gently but firmly sent home. We gave him another date for a week or two later, and he promised himself and us that he would have nothing alcoholic before then to make his visit worthwhile.

When he arrived the next time, he was quite a different person, wide-awake, crisp in his speech and quick in his reactions and responses. His high I.Q. was evident. He looked and felt very much improved.

Walter told us that he had, for some years, been battling with repeated episodes of depression. They were not as black as some people's, but were nonetheless very disagreeable for himself and those around him.

It took the medium only five minutes to pinpoint the facts of Walter's earliest childhood experiences. He had been an illegitimate pregnancy which had caused his parents to get married, though they were not really suited to one another, and did not genuinely love each other. The pregnancy had been a disaster for them both. Therefore, the unborn baby felt he was a disaster. The resultant fear and confusion could only be survived through the development of sustained, life-saving anger. After the birth, the parents continued to see their little one as the unwelcome cause of their unsuitable union. The sensitive boy was aware of their feelings and felt guilty thereafter, though he did not know specifically for what; for existing, he guessed.

He found himself in a quandary. Needing love, he tried to please his parents. However much he tried, they did not acknowledge his efforts but criticised him for any show of rebellion. His rebellion was, unknown to them and the child, simply the result of the anger which had been his survival mechanism and of the totally frustrated search for the parental love and support he had always lacked.

We call this package of deprivation, fear, anger and rebellion infantile despair. The young one feels terrible. Later on, whenever someone or something subconsciously reminds the person of the original situation, up into consciousness comes the original despair and oozes out all over.

Walter, as others like him, had not recognised his depressions as a simple infantile replay, but he could see the point now.

We had no difficulty explaining to him how he had blocked his progress by having alcohol on frequent occasions, although he had never been an alcoholic. He was already aware of man's transcendental nature, having been a student of Buddhist philosophy for some years.

He quickly realised that, by poisoning his brain, he had made it impossible for his own immortal Self to gain dominion over the earthly mechanism. It could, therefore, not control his thought processes and emotions with its love and wisdom. We likened its situation to a driver trying to control a car with a defective transmission and the wrong petrol in the tank. Walter could also see that we were likely to be right when we told him that, in our clinical experience, we had become aware that alcohol was, without a doubt, the single most common cause of depressive episodes in civilised man.

It is about a year at this writing since Walter came to see us. He has kept us informed. He rarely touches alcohol at all now. His marriage, previously teeter-tottering, has stabilised. His wife is happy now. Their two children, who were a bit problematic before, have also calmed down and relaxed. Their performance in school has shown a dramatic upturn. Walter's income has doubled due to his astuteness and presence of mind in his business during the past year.

Walter tells us that, according to his wife, he can be difficult at times, but she now understands how he was traumatised as a child. His states of anger are short- lived now and less and less frequent.

In accordance with our recommendation, Walter has had a frank and open talk with each of his parents separately about the past, about their marriage and its effect on him as a boy. There were some emotional scenes, but Walter insisted that there be honesty between them or no relationship at all. They gave in after a short time and talked, and now the air is clear in the family, and father and mother are also more at peace with one another, a great satisfaction for Walter.

Chapter 12.4 - Success

Paul was sixteen when we first met him and still in school. He was not a brilliant student but passing. A great interest in stock car racing occupied his leisure time. His mother had always proclaimed that Paul would not amount to much because he had been clumsy with his hands from an early age and had no intellectual interests.

Having heard these assertions all his life, Paul was hypnotised by them, especially as his rather learned father, a teacher, did not contradict them at any time. Paul felt at a loose end and floundering in regards to what he might do when he was finished with school. When I asked him more about his current activities he told me rather diffidently that he had recently won a first prize for his work on stock cars and for winning a race.

As soon as I heard this I pointed out to him that he had been brainwashed by his mother's opinion of him, and that he had already completely disproven her ideas. Working with the machines required dexterity and skill and so did driving the winning vehicle.

I said: "Paul, you've been seeing yourself as a loser and you are obviously a winner." He sat and thought for a moment and replied: "By God, you're right. I never thought of it that way." I added: "In fact, you can achieve anything you set your heart on, as you have already shown." Paul: "Right, that does it."

I saw in his face and felt in his being a total shift of gears. Young as he was, Paul thanked me from his heart for his release from bondage.

After finishing school he applied for and obtained a junior management training position in the local branch of a chain store. He had decided he was interested in business. While there, he made sure that he learned not only what was expected of him but all possible angles of buying, selling and merchandising. Being quite a charming personality, Paul had no difficulty in getting the experienced elder personnel to show and teach him what they knew. He quickly formed his own ideas, learning from the mistakes of others as well as from their expertise. He applied himself with the same enthusiasm he had shown for stock car racing.

When he was twenty-one, Paul felt ready to go into business for himself. Borrowing a relatively small sum of money, he took over the franchise for a languishing shop, having satisfied himself that its difficulty lay purely in mismanagement. With amazing speed he turned the business into a fine profit-maker. Equally quickly he repaid his debt. Then he decided to branch out, taking on first one, then still another retail outlet in other locations. Each time he made very sure ahead of time that there was somebody he could trust with the management in his absence as he had to travel between the localities.

For a few years, Paul was "all work and no play", but enjoying his creations. Then he let himself be counselled by friends and employees that he should let up a bit. He bought himself a fine flat near a stock-car race track and paid attention again to his old hobby. Soon he won another event.

He has recently married and will shortly be a father. As of now he feels happy and fulfilled, a self-made man in his twenties.

It was interesting to see what he will do later on in his life. His self-esteem is just fine now. Life will bring him many more challenges. Knowing himself to be a winner now, Paul will probably rise to them.

Chapter 13

Sacrifice case history

Karen's mother had herself had an unhappy childhood from the start. Having received no affection, she became undemonstrative, and to the present day "can't bear physical closeness". She has been an unhappy woman with great guilt feelings. When young, she wanted to pursue an academic career but was unable to finish her education. Married rather young, she had Karen as her first baby. The mother despised her husband for not making a success of his inherited family business, referring to him as a failure ever after. She intended to leave him early on, but remained, ostentatiously, for the sake of the first child which was soon followed by another, a boy.

As the offspring of this embattled couple, Karen could not have been bonded, either prenatally or later. She survived by getting angry. However, this anger could never be expressed at her parents because from the time Karen and her brother were small children, the mother made a number of suicide attempts. Karen well remembers mother frequently asserting that she loved her children. At five years of age Karen consciously realised that if this were true, mother would not wish to abandon them by trying to kill herself. This insight was a great shock for the little girl, one from which she never quite recovered.

Shocks tend to have a hypnotic effect on the individual. So do repetitive traumatic experiences, each confirming the impressions left from the previous one.

Karen's mother also let it be known vociferously that she had "sacrificed" her own interests for the sake of her children. She hated her husband and would always place the children's affairs before his. He was catching his wife's rage against her own father.

Karen sees her father as uncommunicative. His essential stance in the family was a passive one. His own early life was fraught with emotional deprivation. Continuous exposure to his undermining wife kept his self-esteem from rising.

It is an interesting aside that these two now middle-aged people are still living and quarrelling with each other despite there no longer being the excuse of young children.

In Karen's childhood, the mother not only held her husband responsible for her own emotional states, but also made it clear that the children, especially Karen, were to make and keep her happy. She brainwashed them into thinking that they owed her what she had never received from her parents. Consequently, whenever she became self-destructive or simply complained about her unhappiness, Karen immediately felt faulted and guilty. Karen grew up trying to please and appease her mother. Her father was a non-entity as far as the little girl's needs for a strong and loving father were concerned. This was bound to cause Karen endless trouble in her relationships with men later on.

Her identity crisis was obvious when she came to see us upon the recommendation of a friend. Neither parent had given her a positive example. Mother's instability caused the child to find it easier in some ways to imitate father. But that interfered with her essential self-image as a woman.

As Karen got older, Mother made it plain that she expected the girl to accomplish what she herself had failed to do. Karen was to become an academic, to have a career which was bound to bring her a good, safe income and never mind her own preferences.

Karen wanted to do something with her artistic gifts, but that was not allowed. She became a psychiatric social worker. After four years in this profession, she was tired of always dealing with the mentally ill and their families, especially as she tended to take on responsibility that was not rightfully hers. She went into business.

She came to see us about a year after she had started her new work. She felt good about the change she had made, though she still did not feel fulfilled in what she was doing, managing a department with a number of employees under her.

Among other things, the medium told her that much of her difficulty came from the fact that in her last incarnation she had been a nun. Unbonded at that time also, she had said good-bye to ordinary life for her whole adult life. In doing so, she had given up her personal freedom and initiative, and adhered to a system which concerned itself very much with the concepts of sin, guilt, repentance, vicarious responsibility and self-sacrifice. The life was sterile as far as any meaningful self-expression was concerned.

Yet in Ancient Greece Karen had been a dancer, adored by all. She said she still loved to dance, but had done nothing about it.

There had also been a life in Tibet as a man. He was happily married, had children and spent a little time every so often in a nearby monastery as was the custom, bringing any new learning home to wife and family. It was another fulfilled lifetime which had left the memory of a feeling of wholeness and freedom in incarnation deep within the consciousness. The soul would not cease to strive for self-fulfilment.

In Karen's own words: "Part of me feels that I can't do anything right, part knows better than that".

There were two other life-times still influencing Karen now. Both had to do with sacrifice. In one she had been a young Aztec Indian who was chosen for the ritual sacrifice to the Gods which took place every few years in that culture. The young person had no choice in the matter at all, and only the best and most promising individuals were deemed good enough for this dubious honour.

The other experience was when, as the newly bereaved widow of a pharaoh in ancient Egypt, she was ritually walled into a small pyramid, alive, with the deceased pharaoh's entire court, according to custom. On hearing this, Karen exclaimed: "That must be the reason why I've always had a feeling of dread when I'm in a lift and the door closes". She was assured that this symptom would promptly disappear now that she was consciously aware of its origin.

The reader may think that pharaonic Egypt was too long ago to have left such tangible traces in an individual of the twentieth century. Not so! Time, as we experience it, is not what it seems to be. Impressions left in the soul during a life work themselves through and out according to natural law, the law of cause and effect, which makes sure that maximum learning is achieved. It is efficient and precise. No-one and nothing is beyond its beneficent management ever, even for a moment. In our experience, matters not yet resolved are totally current, regardless how old by human reckoning.

This time Karen chose a mother who was bound to remind her of remnant distortions deep in her consciousness regarding sacrifice, being sacrificed and self-sacrifice. A major part of her learning opportunity in the present life would be the recognition of herself as a proud, capable and independent spirit. Saying "no" to her mother's infantile dependency demands on her, and rejecting emotional blackmail firmly with a laugh and with honesty, would be a big step in the right direction, doing both herself and her mother a great deal of good.

Karen must no longer under any circumstances sacrifice her own interests for the sake of other people's emotional satisfaction. It was not for her to take responsibility for other people's decisions, states or errors. At work she would not be able to enjoy herself until she had learned to run her department like a business executive rather than a social worker, straining to make up personally for the deficiencies of employees. She would first need to fall over backwards to run a tight ship.

Her leisure time would have to be spent in her own interest, not sacrificed once again to relatives or others. Her artistic gifts cried out for expression and could be used for her own pleasure and that of others, with possible commercial values firmly in mind. She had to try hard to undo very old habits of feeling that she owed it to others to subject herself to their will, demands and expectations, and of feeling guilty if she did not. She must never let herself be sapped again by others who wished to draw on her energies.

The remaining department in Karen's life which needed a thorough going-over was that of relationships with men. As noted already, the rather vacuous father situation would have left a big gap, an unfilled need in the inner little one combined with an entirely unrealistic picture of what a man, and a woman's personal relationship with him, were all about. These distortions had already taken their toll of Karen's young adult life.

Having involved herself in a sexual affair with a man who was himself trying to satisfy his inner infant, she had become pregnant. Realising the situation was calamitous by this time, Karen opted for a surgical abortion. There were no physical complications but emotionally she suffered greatly once again from guilt feelings, for some time, though knowing that she had done the best she could under the circumstances.

When she came to see us she had recently broken the connection with the man, and felt that she could now get on with her very own life until such time as her love of self, and her self esteem would be so firmly developed that she would no longer relate to a man on the infantile level of needing and then being disappointed; because, as we pointed out to her, until she was quite grown-up herself, she would invariably team up with a much younger soul than herself, in spiritual terms, who was the image of her ineffectual father in one or another respect. Such relationships, common as they are, having nothing whatever to do with genuine love. They are purely on the emotional level, and, being illusory, end up in disaster, whether they last or not. Karen's parents' marriage was a fine illustration of this fact. People who have not experienced true love early on from their parents have first of all to learn to love self, to be at one and at peace with their own spirit before they can fulfil themselves in personal relationships. True adulthood is not about wanting and needing, but about accomplishing and expressing, either alone or together pursuing a spiritual goal in life.

Nature never intended adult sexuality to be used for attempted infantile bonding but as an expression of true love between responsible grown-up people in the spirit of creativity. Seen from the viewpoint of natural, which is also spiritual, law, the wide-spread misuse of sexuality in civilisations is obscene as well as detrimental to the progress of the persons engaged in it.

Although Karen thought she was ready to go her own way for the time being after she had been to see us, her resolve did not last more than a few months. She managed to get herself involved in another affair with an infantile-dependent man for whom she took maternal responsibility. However, she rapidly tired of the situation and has abandoned it, with a firmer resolve this time. It has also taken her some time to stop trying to do her employees' work for them whenever they do not measure up. However, she has learned not to take responsibility for her mother any more. Karen is definitely going forward, though with considerable growing pains so far. It looks as though she will soon relinquish her self-made setbacks. She is tired of her repetitive behaviour.

Lately she has begun to do something about learning to let her fine mediumistic gifts be used by those souls who have stood by her and guided her from another dimension of consciousness. We had recommended a fine teacher for her and for a few others. When these innate gifts are present, they need to be used or the individual suffers from a sense of discontentment and flatness which is often misinterpreted as to its nature.

Karen will be alright. As she gets older, she will use both her talents and her life experience for teaching and treating others in an as yet unknown setting. By then, she will also be an example of positivity for all those who will look to her for help and guidance. At present, she is still undergoing a great and valuable learning in the school of living.

Chapter 14

Readiness

A few weeks before this writing we had a call from a lady whom I shall name Doreen. She identified herself, adding: "You probably don't remember me. I came to see you five years ago. You made me go away again after a short time, telling me that I wasn't ready yet for what you do, and that it would be a waste of my money and your time if I stayed longer. Well, I wasn't ready then, but I am now! I've experienced a lot in the last few years. Many things have happened. Please, can I come back?"

When Doreen came we had a most fruitful session with her. I had looked up the old clinical record and found that we had sent her away because she was what I jokingly call a "butter". This means that whenever one talks about, mentions or suggests is countered by a "Yes, but....". We have learned through experience that nothing constructive comes out of struggling with that attitude. At the time of Doreen's visit five years ago, I was convinced that I had made a mistake in my assessment of her readiness on the telephone before giving her the appointment. After all, errors do happen. However, when I heard Doreen's statement on the phone and the tone of her voice, I realised that the experience of five years ago had a profound impression on her; that it had nurtured the beginning of a new look at life and living.

When we saw her again, there was no childish rebelliousness left. She was quite pleased with herself that she had learned so much from her often painful experiences in the intervening years.

I had given her advice years ago regarding her dietary pattern. She had "but-ted" that also, but did later try it out and found that whenever she complied she felt much better in herself and worse when she fell back into the old self-destructive ways. We had a good laugh with her about these little tales and were able to help her go forward some more.

Last year, a man named Sam came to see us. He behaved worse than Doreen had done. Not only was it "Yes, but ...." at every turn, but he was also obnoxiously and verbosely argumentative, wasting time and energy. We asked him to leave as we had Doreen, but he would not go. We tried several times. He shook his head and stayed glued to his chair. We told him that there was no sense in continuing with him in this state. He said: "I have come a long way, travelled several hours. I've got to make it worth my while." We said we would continue to work with him if he changed his behaviour.

All this took only a few minutes. Sam said he would now cooperate, and so he did. We had a worthwhile session with him and Sam left a great deal more grown-up than he had come in. He would never again be the same. He had, in fact, been able to laugh at his childish behaviour.

I have cited these two people, Doreen and Sam, because they and a few others like them have taught us that, working under inspiration, we sometimes make what we think are mistakes. Yet the experience is giving patients precisely the opportunity needed to be able to turn a corner in their state of being.

I now call these situations "shock treatments". They are far from easy for ourselves, yet obviously worth-while from the viewpoint of the spirit when the recipient of the shock is destined to make a real contribution to human progress once matured.

Section III

The Pioneer -

Lisa Sand MD

Chapter 15

Early Adventures

Born in 1922 in Germany, I grew up in the Nazi period from the age of eight. Hitler took absolute power when I was nine. I despised what was going on from its very beginnings as I witnessed its results in school and among the population in general. In 1939, aged sixteen, I had the opportunity to go to England where I arrived just three weeks before the outbreak of the Second World War.

It had been arranged that I would fly from Munich to London in August 1939. Commercial planes were small and very slow then, landing frequently. They hardly compared with today's jet airliners. I remember looking out of the window at take-off, seeing my parents getting smaller and smaller as I set off into an uncertain future with my ticket and the permitted £3 in my pocket.

A few tears later, I turned my thoughts to how I would behave at the check-point in Frankfurt airport where I was to change to a Dutch airline for the flight to London. That last contact with the German authorities behind me, I felt a tremendous relief when we were airborne again and finally crossed the border. There would be no more Nazi Germany for me. This feeling of liberation outweighed my sorrow at leaving my parents, possibly forever.

My earliest memory is that of lying on my back in a white-lined baby cot, my arms and legs moving. Two smiling faces looked down at me from above, one from each side. They were my parents. I felt cheerfully excited, knowing I was the cause of their pleasure.

From that fleeting memory of my own, I go to one of my mother's, told me many years later. When I was old enough to sit in a high chair and she had work to do in the kitchen, she would give me a teaspoon to play with. I would make a thorough-going study of this object in its various aspects and possibilities for a long time, in utmost concentration. She realised that my attention span and focussed investigation were unusual for a baby. She tried me out time and again with the same result.

Though the objects and subjects of my studies later on were not table silver, I have not changed a bit in this respect.

Throughout my young years, while my playmates' hands and clothes had to be cleaned up more or less forcibly, I would come into the house and ask to have my hands washed and clothes tidied. I remember disliking the feeling of being soiled in any way. My mother complied, silently astonished at my attitude. Little did she or I realise that in my last life before the present one, I was greatly concerned with the then young science of bacteriology and had worked at trying to teach matters of public hygiene to people in a backward part of the world.

I developed a burning interest in bacteriology and immunology in my late teens. I was twenty before I had enough training in the basic sciences of chemistry and biology to be eligible for these studies. I undertook them then with real gusto, rapidly adding some undergraduate research projects with the encouragement of my professors.

These extra activities consumed most of my spare time. The research meant delving into the unknown in a disciplined fashion, and I loved every minute of it. It was all my own doing with advice given only upon my request. The years were 1943 to 1945. The world was at war in Europe and in the Pacific. I felt strangely unreal at Smith College in Northampton, Massachusetts, U.S.A., as if on a peaceful island in a troubled sea. My intense interest in bacteriology seemed completely out of sync with my firm intention to study medicine and specialise in psychiatry later. Little did I know that it was my last incarnation's professional expertise which caused my inner self to want to catch up with developments in its former speciality in the decades since its departure from planet Earth!

To the astonishment of my parents I spoke well enough to express my meaning at the age of one year. I do, in fact, distinctly remember the pleasure I had when I could communicate verbally with the people around me from that time on, and I expected to have my statements taken seriously. There was, for instance, the time when my mother had sat me in my pram in front of the house. I remember that she looked up at the sky and decided that she ought to go back upstairs to get something. A small group of children was playing on the pavement. My mother spoke to them about guarding the pram with me in it and they were very willing. As soon as she had disappeared into the house, they started to squabble about which of them was to hold onto the handle of the pram and push it around. I quite disliked the conflict, sat myself up to full height and took charge, saying I would make the decisions. All the children quietened down and I remember pointing to first one then another to take turns. It could have been only a matter of seconds before my mother returned to an entirely peaceful scene. I felt very pleased with myself. The incident revived ancient memories of a self-image as a natural leader and peace-maker.

However, the early speech development did not always work out to advantage. I remember sitting in my pram being pushed across the cobble-stoned central square of the town. A tall man holding an Alsation dog on a leash came towards us. He took his hat off and greeted my mother who spoke to him in return. Though I was extremely interested in the dog I heard the conversation. I remember saying something to the man whereupon his expression changed completely and he rapidly took his leave, to my disappointment. My mother pushed the pram away equally quickly, clearly agitated. I was mystified as I had only tried to make my presence known by impressing the man with my knowledge.

Many years later I learned that I had said to him "My parents say that you are a milksop!". The man was the Chief of Police. My father and mother were glad to move to another town a few months later. They also determined not to talk about other people undisguised within earshot of their little hazard for years to come. Though I could not understand what had gone wrong, I became aware of the power of the word in an undesirable direction. The world was an interesting place.

The time when I was one year of age was one of rich experience. The following is another which I remember with crystal clarity. In the flat below us lived the owners of the terraced house. I was very friendly with the lady, "Auntie Anna", who often cooked broth from bones and would give me a bone to gnaw when it was cool enough. She had a son who would have been about fourteen or fifteen years old. I had a crush on him. When he paid attention to me I was in seventh heaven.

One day when the son was home, I was momentarily alone with him in his parents' living room. Though obviously quite capable of walking, I had been refusing to do so unless I could hold onto a piece of furniture or somebody's hand. I remember standing in a corner of the room. The young man, keeping up a running conversation with me, slowly walked backwards towards the opposite corner. While I was transfixed by his attention he beckoned me to come to him. I ran to him. No sooner arrived, I realised that he had tricked me. A murderous howl on my part was the result. His mother came running from the kitchen, mine from upstairs. Never could I forget the scene of the two women trying to understand what was going on. I screeched furiously, the young man looked gratifyingly sheepish as he tried to explain what had happened above my din.

I had adored him. From now on, as he had wounded my pride so deeply, I would disdain him even if it hurt me too. However, having inadvertently demonstrated that I could walk alone, I henceforth did, judging it wiser to give in on that point.

My first passionate affair of the heart had ended in betrayal. It was not to be the last one.

Despite the emotional shock of the experience just recounted, I had to admit to myself that walking and running increased my freedom of action substantially. I enjoyed that. In the hallway of my parents' flat was a prominent cupboard which contained all the household linen. I had observed this to be of particular importance during the weekly visit of the cleaning lady. Next time she came through the front door I was there with my mother to receive her. I took her by a finger and pulled her to the linen cupboard. With my free hand I pointed up to it and said "This is mine". To this day I remember her slightly startled and bemused expression. Having stated my case so emphatically I let go of her and set about my business feeling very satisfied with myself and the world.

While I was a babe in arms my mother would take me for a daily stroll in my pram as was the custom, weather permitting. She soon noticed that, whenever she turned in a homeward direction, I vociferously objected. She quietly began to experiment with me, taking the pram through various streets in different directions and on a variety of pathways through the park-like cemetery nearby. I would still begin to object as soon as she headed home. She could never figure out how I could possible recognise the way, different each time, lying in the carriage.

Though I later remembered parts and pieces of several lifetimes as a North American Indian, I feel that path-finding by observation and an excellent sense of direction were not the explanation. I am sure that I psychically received her intention to go home. After all, who has not known an animal, especially a dog, pick up its master's unspoken thought of going for a walk? Thought transference is the most basic communication between all creatures, as is foreknowledge of conditions. A vixen who has her young in a burrow on the side of a river will seek a more elevated home for them and carry them to safety shortly before a flood occurs. All of nature is thought and the uncluttered consciousness perceives with ease what is "hidden from the wise".

Very soon after I started to walk on my own, I was taken on one of our regular visits to the home of two ladies who were friends of my parents. My latest accomplishment was duly admired. But as I demonstrated it I came across a most disagreeable obstacle. I still see it looming dangerously before me. It was the raised wooden doorstep which I had to negotiate to get into the next room. The door was wide open. Having run up to this point, I stopped dead with my left hand on the door joist. The more I stared at the monster before me the bigger it became. However, I was simply not going down on all fours to cross it. While I stood there I remember hearing coaxing female voices behind me, and felt an urge within me to overcome the fear and take the chance.

Somehow I was aware that the thing seemed very much worse than it was. Though I have no clear recollection, I do believe I managed to negotiate it by myself.

I was then and am still cautious about assorted physical dangers. I am keen on accident prevention for the population as a whole. Disregard of safety measures and wanton carelessness are guaranteed to arouse my indignation.

The town in which I was born is in the Rhineland. During the time I lived there it was French occupied territory following the First World War. Occupational forces were everywhere. As a tiny one I was very eager for the shiny buttons on the French officers' uniforms. My mother was worried about my loud clamouring for these bright objects in passing but not once did any of the officers feel offended by the baby's expression of demand. Neither, of course, did I ever obtain one of the coveted things. Even at my present advanced age I am still fascinated by anything that sparkles, glitters or shines brightly, regardless of its intrinsic value or the lack of it. Am I secretly still reaching for the French officers' buttons?

While I was still a toddler my parents and I moved to the nearby city of Aachen (Aix-la-Chapelle). There we were again in a first-floor flat. On the ground floor lived a doctor with his wife and several children, two of them of an age compatible with mine. That was fine. Having no brother or sister of my own, I always wanted to be in the company of children and my parents tried to live where this need of mine could be met. Frankly, I am sure that I would have been completely unbearable if I could not have had a social life of my own. Adults were terribly boring most of the time.

From our flat a very narrow winding staircase led to the attic which was used for storage. The door at the head of the stairs was kept locked and I was not allowed to go up on my own.

Therefore, it seemed to me that there was a mysterious world of hidden treasure up there, and I remember looking up those curving steps, either longing to delve into that secret world or half enjoying the mystery for its own sake. Forbidden fruit is very attractive.

Whenever in my life I have visited an old castle or a tower with a winding stairway, I have climbed it with an inner senses of excitement and anticipation of what I would find at the top.

The younger children downstairs in our new abode, though available, were on the whole disappointingly dull. The older ones spent most of their time at school, and I am sure that I was just too young to be of real interest to them. Nonetheless, I worked out some simple games I could play with the smaller ones, especially in the enclosed courtyard of the building where our mothers could see and hear us with ease. I still remember the aspect of the cobble-stones from a sharp angle as my eyes were not far above their surface.

My father attached a swing for me on the wooden joist above a door in the flat. I felt grateful for this gift of love. Even today I enjoy a swing when I come across one which matches my present size and weight.

Shortly after my sixth birthday, my father and I stood at a window where we had put food out for the birds as the ground was covered with snow. My father, a very tall man, looked down at me fondly and with a wistful expression on his face said "If I had had a son, I would have wanted him to become a doctor".

This statement shot like an arrow into my heart. Immediately I put two and two together and felt that my father would have preferred a boy and could not see a girl fulfilling his dream. My whole inner self revolted instantaneously and I silently vowed "I'll show you! I will become a physician".

Maybe it required this painful experience to make sure that I would actually pursue the course that was meant for me without wavering, despite the fact that there was not a single doctor or scholar of any kind in my whole extended clan. Twenty years later, in Philadelphia, Pa., U.S.A., I received the degree of Doctor of Medicine, capped and gowned as is the custom to this day. By that time I had long realised that this and no other was the desired career for me, quite aside from my father's thoughts. He had died seven years before my graduation. In fact, I never saw him again after I left Germany at sixteen.

Chapter 16

Glimpses of Reality

When I was about seven years old I sat at table with my parents as usual in the kitchen. It must have been winter because it was pitch-dark outside at supper-time. We lived at that time at the very edge of the city of Regensburg on the bank of the Danube. Having no neighbours, my parents had not drawn the curtains. They sat across from each other, talking; I faced the black window. Suddenly I jumped up, staring. My father asked what had happened. I pointed outside and told him that a huge face had appeared just beyond the glass. However, it had not been a human face. It was like an oversized full moon. In a moment it was gone again.

The experience had startled me. My parents looked out across the fenced-in garden and the large garden next to it. There was nothing and no-one to see. An investigation next day showed that no-one had been outside in either property that evening. Many years would go by before I was to realise that this was a clairvoyant episode having to do with a greatly beloved soul I had known in a life when he and I were both American Indians and his name had been "Silver Moon".

Between the ages of six and nine years I had a number of repetitive psychic experiences in the night.

In one, I was in a little child's body facing a half-circle of robed figures all looking down at me with lively interest. I knew they were close and loving friends and that I had made plans and agreements with them whose nature I could no longer fathom. The scene was one of a cheerful goodbye. I turned and ran to a large round opening and carried on determinedly right into it. Instead of falling downward, I was floating. The feeling was an uncomfortable one, but not frightening. The shaft was quite dark but nearing the bottom I could see it dimly lit. I floated right on down and landed in something soft like a net. Next I was lying in a baby bassinet as a newborn, with my parents looking down at me, smiling.

Again, though somewhere I had an inkling, many years passed before I realised that this had not been a dream, but a recollection of the process of incarnation. And there was the realisation that I had an agreed purpose for the incarnation, that I was a member of an enterprising, loving team of collaborators and friends in the dimension of ultimate reality.

In the other repetitive "dream" I was pure individual consciousness looking from close range at a greyish-beige homogeneous muddy mass moving in swirls, one next to the other, a dizzy-making rather unpleasant image as I got still closer. The next thing I experienced was waking up in my bed. Often I felt considerable resistance to getting so close to this mass or mess. However, at times the swirls reflected light in rainbow colours, like a very thin layer of oil on a puddle of water. Then it was much more cheerful and interesting, but I still found the approach difficult when I got very close.

This "dream" recurred once or twice at a much later age also. I have since realised that the swirling mass was matter itself as seen from another dimension of consciousness: muddy swirls of energy in a state of negativity, brightly coloured when positive. Sometimes it was partly muddy, partly reflecting colour. In the night, in what we call deep sleep, I had been out of my body and gone home. Then I came back for another day on earth and had to enter the illusion which is the world of matter, including the body I am using called Lisa.

I know that I am not in my body in deep sleep. Nonetheless, I do not and did not usually remember my temporary exits and re-entries on awakening. That is a good thing because the entry was not the most pleasant of experiences while I was a child. Yet I seem to have learned to do it much more smoothly and also more rapidly now. I remember once, not very long ago, being in the company of friends or colleagues in the dimension of reality and realising that I simply had to return to my body during the night to remove the duvet which covered it before it got too hot. There was much laughter all around about this quick but necessary job as I set off with a quip. On a number of occasions I have had to come back and adjust the body's position because it was getting into considerable trouble snoring, with the tongue so deeply relaxed that the body was partly choking while lying on its back. As I got into the body I became aware that the condition was similar to that of surgical anaesthesia. But as no drug was involved, the physical distress signal registered with the soul which immediately returned to take care of its vehicle. The adjustment made, it was off again.

On awakening in the morning I only remember the quick re-entry, the adjustment and determinedly leaving again because I was busy elsewhere. What these activities in another dimension are about is evidently not the concern of my daytime consciousness as the memory would surely distract me from my business on earth. Such distraction would be counter-productive. My earthly self understands that and acquiesces without probing or demanding to know. I am aware that every demand by the human personality to fathom conditions in other dimensions not only leads to gross errors but also causes distress and alarm to the soul. The material intellect is of extremely limited capacity. It is of constructive use only when directly under the loving dominance and direction of the spirit.

At the age of twelve I read the book *"The Last Days of Pompeii"*. I found it an interesting and entertaining novel until I came to the very last page on which the author dealt with the actual eruption of Vesuvius. Suddenly I found myself, about twelve years old, standing at the pointed end of a large, gaily decorated wooden ship facing Pompeii, my home. The sea was calm. Within a second there was nothing but a impenetrably dense cloud of something like dust before me where the shore had been, accompanied by a roar. As I stood there, rigid with terror, I heard another sound close by: here and there a stone fell into the water, so hot that it created hissing steam as it entered the sea. Not one fell into the ship.

I do not remember the story of the novel. At age twelve and after I could not explain the strange first-hand experience just described. Many years were to pass before I realised that this was a memory rather than a fantasy. As a middle-aged woman I became acquainted with a couple of other people who had been on that same ship with me in Roman times. They also remembered.

A year later I walked into a room with a television set. On the screen was a view of the ash coming down from the volcano erupting in the state of Washington in the Northwestern United States at the time. Again I stood transfixed, looking at the screen. A very unpleasant ripple or current of a quasi-physical sensation ran through my entire being and then was gone, never to return, regardless how many more news-views of the same sort of scene I saw. It was clear to me that it had required the broadcast to remove the last vestiges of the shock still remaining in the soul two thousand years after the event.

What is time?

At the age of twelve I made up my mind to emigrate to the U.S.A. at the earliest possible opportunity. The year was 1935, the Nazis firmly in control of Germany. Though I had never been out of Germany, not even for a day, I was deeply disgusted with what was going on. My parents, always respecting my life decisions, placed no obstacles in my way. My mother, in fact, did her very best to help me achieve my goal as time passed and war grew more and more imminent. However, despite the efforts of a cousin in America, I could not obtain a visa to the United States. Meanwhile, in the spring of 1939, a distant relative in London managed to secure a "permit" to England for me. On the 9th August 1939 I set off for London from Munich airport.

In the late autumn of 1939 a German-speaking Czechoslovakian lady, who had managed to escape to England before the Germans annexed her country, was staying in the same place as I was. She had a small framed photograph of herself, a man and a little girl on her night-table. I asked her who the other two were. She said "The man is my husband, the girl is my daughter". I looked her straight in the eye as I said "Your husband is not the father of your child". She jumped out of her seat, completely startled. "How did you know that, how could you know that? I've never told anyone but an old friend in Switzerland years ago!". I went away rapidly, leaving her in a state of considerable consternation.

But what about me? I had no concept or knowledge of mediumship. Yes, how did I know what I had so calmly and confidently stated? Now I also was in a state of turmoil, almost afraid of myself. But I was young and soon got over it. So very much was happening and needed to be done.

At sixteen going on seventeen, I was the youngest inhabitant in that environment of women who ranged all the way into their sixties. All of us were temporarily quartered in a small boarding school in North London. The pupils and teachers had been evacuated. There was a woman of twenty-six with a round face and exceedingly red cheeks. She had come from Austria, the first independent country to be annexed by the Nazis. She always seemed to feel ill and unhappy and made no secret of it. She and I had a joint chore to do in the kitchen. Whenever we worked together she took the opportunity to beg me to come to see her where we could be alone. As I did not find her company interesting, I resisted. Then one day, when no-one was listening, she said "I don't know why it is. You are so much younger than I am but whenever you have been with me I feel very much better for some time".

This gave me something to think about. I knew nothing about spirit healing, had never heard of such a thing. I had felt somehow that this lady's difficulties, whatever physical component or expression there might have been, were from her emotions and her thoughts. Reflecting on this extraordinary set of circumstances, I made a decision: not only would I become a doctor but I would then specialise in psychiatry.

How all this ambition was to be realised was a total unknown. I did not mention it to anyone because I knew other people would laugh at such ideas on the part of a penniless displaced young person. But I was sure that my notions were not youthful fantasies. Though I knew nothing of the spirit on the outer level, its feelings and intentions found access to my daytime consciousness.

My future looked dim in wartime Britain and my heart still longed for the U.S.A. which loomed brightly to me as the "land of opportunity". My cousin there had managed to get a full scholarship for me at an Episcopal (English Church) girls' convent school in the state of Kentucky. He had applied for me through the Friends' (Quaker) Service Committee in New York and I had been selected because I had been a pupil in German convent schools, as a boarder and as a day student, for several years although I was a Protestant. The scholarship had been granted in the spring and I had not been able to obtain any kind of visa to enter the U.S.A. The nuns in Kentucky had appealed to Mrs Eleanor Roosevelt, wife of President Roosevelt. She had written to Ambassador Joseph Kennedy, father of the future President, on my behalf. He had replied to her rather testily, setting out in detail the portion of the immigration law of the United States which showed unequivocally that my category of applicant was not entitled to any kind of visa other than under the quota system. The quota, as it applied to me, was packed out for at least ten years ahead. "Sorry, Mrs Roosevelt!".

This last letter, being of such finality, should have caused the nuns in Kentucky and me to give the matter up as a lost cause. Neither party did. The nuns prayed for a miracle and I went to try once again to get into the U.S. Consulate in Grosvenor Square, London, though I had never yet got past the doorman. This time was no exception. An acquaintance met me outside the building and asked me to tea. First I had to go back with her to the office where she worked, while she finished some filing begun earlier. There, as I was waiting for her, a customer of one of the young lady's employers began a conversation with me. It evolved rapidly that this gentleman and his family had come from the same German city where I had lived and that he had been friendly with a U.S. consular official there who was now working at the embassy in Grosvenor Square. The gentleman said "I would like to help you get a visa. Meet me in front of the main entrance of the Consulate on Wednesday morning at ten o'clock".

Meet me there he did, right on time. As we walked towards the door he gave me a few simple instructions on how to behave, when to talk and when not. He showed his card to the doorman and we both walked in with ease where I had not been permitted to set foot all the times I had tried. Less than an hour later we walked out again with a legally valid American visa in my passport.

My benefactor, whose name was a household word in Munich, walked a part of the way with me. There was a beggar on the pavement. With a dramatic flourish Mr 'X' dropped a sizeable coin into the beggar's hat to celebrate the success of our venture. Then he asked me if I would post a letter to his sister in New York when I arrived in the United States. It was wartime and transatlantic post was not reliable. British ships were being torpedoed by German U-boats. Both of us felt that I would be safe and therefore the letter with me.

I was dancing on air. Immediately I made my way to the refugee aid committee in charge of my case. When I walked in announcing that I had a U.S. visa the two case workers looked at me pityingly, as if to say "There's another one gone crazy". One of them languidly told me to give her my passport. When I did, she was speechless. As soon as she was able to speak again, she exclaimed to the other lady "It's true!".

I was having fun watching them as they momentarily both doubted their own reason.

Passage was arranged there and then on one of the very last British ships transporting civilian passengers across the Atlantic. On Christmas Eve I left from Liverpool, one of fifty civilian passengers aboard a small old Cunard Line freighter. After an adventurous journey of nearly three weeks I landed in Boston. It was January 1940. Almost two years were to pass before the United States declared war on Japan and Germany.

Studying medicine and then specialising in psychiatry remained my educational goal. Though I had the above-mentioned full scholarship in Kentucky to obtain a High School diploma, there were no financial means for going to a university. When I stayed at the school at the beginning of the summer holiday, a retreat was held there to which an old friend of the Mother Superior came. This lady was then studying medicine in Boston. The Reverend Mother told her about me and her friend became very interested. She went for a walk with me and asked me about my plans for the future. Ascertaining that I did not have the means to go the way I wished, she asked me how I intended to get them.

I said I would work my way through the required eight years of training, even if I had to take considerably longer in order to earn the necessary money in between. Just then our walk was finished and we entered the building.

Next day the retreat was over and the participants left for home. In the afternoon the Reverend Mother called me into her office, sat me down and then said that Frances, her friend, had told her to let me know that she would pay for my further education so that I would not have to add extra years in order to support myself. Frances was wealthy enough to do this.

Once again, I felt propelled mysteriously in my chosen direction. I was very grateful indeed and thought deeply about what had happened to me during the preceding two years. Mathematically it did not make much sense. Each successive event, by the law of averages, had a chance of one in several thousand to one in a million or more. Added together, the chances reached near impossibility, especially in such rapid succession.

I felt distinctly that there was no coincidence in any of the events but an infinitely intelligent, deliberate management which elegantly swept aside improbability and even apparent impossibility.

My head was spinning. I was at the receiving end of something unfathomably beautiful, powerful, warm and loving. Once again I had this feeling of a greater reality. Briefly, I sensed the world as unreal. Knowing there was no-one who would understand, I kept these impressions to myself.

Chapter 17

Responsibilities

Following my graduation from High School in 1941 I went to Berea College, Kentucky, for two years. Then I received a full scholarship to the prestigious Smith College in Northampton, Massachusetts, where I graduated with honours in 1945. The next step was the Medical College of Pennsylvania, at that time called "The Women's Medical College of Pennsylvania". Another four years later, in 1949, I graduated as a Doctor of Medicine.

1949 was significant for yet another reason. Shortly after beginning my internship in a busy city-centre hospital, I met a senior medical student, six years older than I, and married him six weeks later. As I only had one and a half days off every two weeks, we were married on a Saturday afternoon. On the Saturday morning I found myself having to do an autopsy all alone as the pathologist, knowing of my plans for the afternoon, took his time coming in to relieve me. I believe he, a married man in his forties, was jealous. He nearly made me late for my wedding but he could not prevent it.

It took another nine months before my husband and I could actually live together. The hospital in which I worked is in a city located sixty miles from Philadelphia where he was in his last year of medical school. By the time we set up house together our first child was on the way. There were two more to follow. For me as a mother, special training in psychiatry was somewhat interrupted and spread out in time as I wanted to raise the little ones myself. In retrospect, the life experience I gained from doing so was immensely valuable, right to the present day. No amount of professional experience could have substituted for it.

Regardless how much time I spent with the children while they were small, I was never out of touch with my chosen profession because my husband had also specialised in psychiatry. We learned from and with each other. It was marvellous to be able to talk it all over at will and at leisure.

When the time came for me to set up my own practice, I soon changed it to include a number of very important aspects of scientifically-based but unusual types of what I might now call "holistic" medicine. I had used much of my spare time making a study of these things, realising that a healthy body and a resilient, capable stress mechanism were essential for the achievement and maintenance of a healthy mind. "Mens sana in corpore sano" - a healthy mind in a healthy body. In contrast to my husband, I did not care for the use of drugs to influence mood or behaviour. These medications mushroomed out of the pharmaceutical industry in the years after our training. I shied away from any long-term artificial or manipulative intervention with the human consciousness, though I did not clearly know why in those days.

Chapter 18

A Re-awakening

The differences of opinion in regards to the way my husband and I each practiced medicine did not cause any friction between us. But by and by other matters led to a parting of the ways after nearly twenty-eight years. Not least among them was the fact that, after a particularly harsh blow of "fate" which hit both of us, we reached the point where not only he but I too felt that I was at my wit's end in regard to dealing with it.

I was standing in the living room by myself, looking out at a range of mountains, clearly saying in my mind: "If there be a God, may He help me now. I have gone as far as I can." Then I let go of thinking and went about my daily business.

I had arranged a meeting with a young patient who had come two thousand miles to seek my help and had progressed wonderfully in a very short time. While I was with him he brought out a book which had been loaned to him by another young patient who had not had the courage to show it to me.

Would I please take a look at it and tell him what I thought of it. Its title was "*The Sleeping Prophet*". I read what was printed on the jacket and said: "This is all completely new to me. I can't possibly make any judgement without having actually read the book. Can I take it with me?" The young man looked very relieved and delighted.

"*The Sleeping Prophet*" was the first published biography of the well-known American trance medium Edgar Cayce. I had never heard of him. Over the next couple of days I read the book. A whole new world opened up for me. I told both of my young patients that it all made sense to me. A feeling of joy and adventure filled me. I remember scouring the public library for further literature on similar subjects and there finding the so-called "Betty books", a whole series written by Stuart E. White about his wife, Betty, who had been a fine trance medium. After her "death" she used an old friend as her own trance medium, supplying Stuart with information to publish. Some of it was of great interest to open-minded scientists of that time.

Shortly after becoming acquainted with these realities of the unseen world about us and its loving comradeship I started to travel to Europe. For twenty-eight years I had not left North America. In London I found places where I could make appointments to see experienced mediums. I took as much advantage of the situation as I could, also attending a number of lectures and acquiring some literature.

Altogether I felt that I had come home, as my heart sang to have rediscovered a lost world and friends of long ago. While I was in London my own mediumship and spiritual healing ability were pointed out to me repeatedly. Indeed, back in the U.S. it was not long before these things were proved to me in daily life, both at home and in my medical practice.

Painful was the reception my enthusiasm received from the two adults most closely associated with me. My husband, though he had no trouble proving his own healing mediumship to himself and others, was frightened and became sarcastic and undermining. My mother, living only a short distance away, had long wished me to be just an ordinary run-of-the-mill respected and contented medical practitioner instead of the pioneer I had become. While she and my husband gave vent to the dissatisfactions, they had for years been very willing to profit personally from my new techniques and harmless but effective treatments. The improvements in their own health suited them well, and the children had also profited. Going further ahead into uncharted waters in this atmosphere of opposition was a lonely business indeed. But my destiny was pulling at me, whatever the odds might be.

Within two years of reading *"The Sleeping Prophet"* it was clear to me that my time in America was over, though I had had no wish to go elsewhere for three decades. My husband also found himself enamoured of Europe, although for different reasons. We settled in Germany where the two younger children could be integrated scholastically into a private school with relative ease. We lived on the Alpine border, very near Austria. Within a short time I was able to practice medicine again.

However, I continued to long for England and kept up my connections there, visiting two to four times a year.

Three times during those few years I had remarkable experiences during the night while my body lay in the sleep state. They were very different from dreams and gave me much to think about. Again, my communications about these events and their significance were ill-received. The gap between my husband and me became ever wider.

Although all my remembered excursions into another dimension of consciousness were breathtaking, one in particular deserves to be recounted here.

I had left my physical body asleep. The spiritual body which was I did not look like the already middle-aged woman in bed in Bavaria. I was young, very young and slender, a "slip of a thing" in a rather long white dress of a soft draping fabric, sleeveless and round-necked. It looked very much like the gowns depicted on ancient Greek statues and images. A softly-gathered bodice was joined to an equally gathered skirt at the waist, held by a simple belt or cord. Gold-blonde curly locks of hair were crowned by a golden diadem. I was this figure and at the same time I could see myself as it.

Knowing exactly where I was going, without a thought in my head, I moved rapidly, arriving at a beautiful entrance door guarded by a being not dissimilar to myself. We communicated by thought. To my questioning look the guard asked me to wait just a little. Then the door opened wide. I entered a great hall where three tall beings stood on the raised platform, the tallest between the other two. They looked around at me as I quickly walked to the front of the platform, facing them.

I knelt down while a great love welled up in my heart as I looked at the central figure with the words "Mein Vater, Mein König!" - "My Father, my King". He took a long flat object in his right hand, touched my left shoulder with it once, then, turning it round, touched it with the other side. Just as quickly, I was on my feet again. During this ceremony there was the most beautiful singing of a large chorus ranged in groupings, tier above tier, on my right. The sound was crystal clear, the sopranos higher than any I have ever heard on earth.

Standing there briefly, bathed in love, I received the thought from my initiator to return to earth to carry out the task which was mine. As I walked back towards the door I turned round, beaming the question whether I might know on earth what the task was. The initiator shook his head. I walked out then and found myself back in my physical body, awake in an instant. Try as I would, I could not remember the faces or exact aspects of the three figures on the platform. But I was deeply impressed by the experience as well as puzzled. My earthly mind quickly remembered the mediaeval ceremony of knighting. I realised that what had happened in the night was the original of which knighting is a distorted copy. The spatula-like tool had nothing to do with the sword used by man on earth. Another thing which astonished me was my graceful, matter-of-course compliance with the ceremony. On earth I was not a lover of pageantry.

I could see the reason for my prejudice: Most earthly rites and pageants were just blindly repeated custom. The original, deeply spiritual meaning had been lost, leaving the door wide open to material superficiality and even misuse.

As indicated by the initiator, back in my body I could not fathom what my task was, yet I had always known I had one.

Chapter 19

"Lost" and Found

One morning in 1972 I awoke early. The word "Universitas" kept repeating in my mind. I liked the sound of it, the lilt of the syllables pronounced in Latin. I knew that it was a concept, a living, learning and teaching of cosmic truth, the universal law of cause and effect. There was in me a great longing and a great love for the kind of people who could and would collaborate in such an undertaking with all their hearts and minds. The wisdom and devotion for such an enterprise could not come easily. It would require the closest cooperation between the unseen world and the material world. Much would have to be very ancient, and some entirely new. The concept had engraved itself deeply into my consciousness. As the years passed and the home situation deteriorated, I kept recalling the idea to mind. Each time it steadied me. Fantastic as it might seem, somehow I had to steer towards it.

My practice in Bavaria increased rapidly as my reputation spread. Before long I had a number of patients for whom I would have liked the services of a reliable medium to work with me. I could not find one in Germany or Austria. The need for such help felt more and more acute. I decided to look for a British-trained German-speaking medium in London through the three largest organisations there. My hunt proved fruitless. However, never having been one for giving up easily, I tried again on my next visit. Again, no-one knew of any German-speaking medium. I felt frustrated and a bit sad.

As I was already in the building of one of the organisations, I asked if there was a seat to be had in a group session with any of their mediums right then and there. A lady at the reception desk looked up the roster and said "This is strange. We have precisely one opening and that is with Inga Hooper. She is usually fully booked weeks ahead of time." I had never met Inga Hooper. As I was one of five or six people in her group, she only spent ten minutes on me personally. Everything she told me was correct and interesting. Then she said "I have a man here by the name of Keitel." She pronounced the German name "Keetel". "There is something familiar about that name but I cannot place it".

She thought intently but then shook her head. Meanwhile I assured her that I knew exactly who that was. He had in fact become a friend of ours when we first moved to Germany and had since died. His name was familiar to her because he had been a first cousin of the famous Field Marshall Keitel. Pronouncing the name "Keetel" instead of the German way "Ky-tel" did not seem strange to me for an English person.

When the meeting was over, all the participants left the room. I saw Mrs Hooper starting down the stairs while I was crowded into the little lift with the others. As the lift started down, a man said to his wife "How strange that Mrs Hooper didn't recognise that name? Isn't she Austrian?" I was electrified. "Did you say Austrian?" "Yes; or is it German?"

No way could that lift be stopped till it reached the street level. I got out, ran up the stairs at top speed and met Inga Hooper just outside the Ladies' room. I spoke to her in German and she answered in kind. What joy!

As I had to fly back home the next morning and she had another session to do, we quickly arranged to meet in the cafeteria half an hour later, during her tea-break. The time seemed endless and then the two of us sat across from each other and talked. I told her of my prolonged hunt and she could not understand why none of the people I had asked seemed to know of her Austrian and German background. She had never kept if a secret. We decided that I should have enquired from head office rather than reception. But maybe it was just that the time had not been right sooner.

Looking back at both of our lives in those years, I am sure that neither of us would have been ready earlier for what was to follow. Guidance from another dimension made sure that we did not meet too soon. After all, our own higher consciousness knew its goal, even though the "sleepy" earth mind had but a dim realisation of it.

Starting while I was still living in the United States, I had had a marked longing to work with a reliable medium on suitable patients, though circumstances there would have prohibited me from doing any such thing. Inga Hooper meanwhile had known psychically for many years that one day she would work with a lady doctor; in what capacity, she had no idea.

Some time after our meeting, Inga Hooper came to Germany to help me with the patients I had lined up for the privilege. Every single one of them was immensely grateful for the insights and clarification received through our combined effort. The two of us felt a great sense of satisfaction from working together in this fashion. We also found that we enjoyed each other's company and interests. Over a period of two years we repeated the experiment several times, always with the same success.

It became more and more clear to me that my true goal, that of Universitas, lay in the direction of our work together. To this end I had to make some very tough personal decisions, letting go of emotional attachments and conventional thinking. Aware that all dis-ease is rooted in the soul, I would have to change course and embark full-time and with complete devotion on my new enterprise of research.

Inga Hooper and I were obviously destined to work together. Britain offered the greatest amount of freedom for the carrying-out of our plan.

It took another year for me to free myself so completely that I was able to join Inga in England to begin a new and different life.

Having left our respective personal pasts behind us with determination, we set our to follow our innermost convictions as to what health and disease - or dis-ease - are really all about. The combination of a scientific background, internal medicine and psychiatric practice on the one hand, and highly disciplined mediumship on the other including teaching, gave us the tools as well as the courage to be pioneers. Our combined professional experience in our respective fields already totalled about seventy years. Our personal life experience covered a valuable one hundred and twenty five years added together. In my view there is no substitute for the latter which I refer to as the University of Living. It does not issue a paper diploma but the opportunity to acquire deeply-abiding knowledge to be drawn on ever after. Instant empathy, an automatic sympathetic understanding of the state of being of others, must have such a foundation. Fortunately, it is an on-going process which, though it can be resisted, cannot be arrested.

Over a period of about ten years I had been told by a number of mediums that I would one day write a book or books, something I had never considered. When I had joined Inga in England, the soul whom we earthlings last knew in incarnation as Professor Carl Gustav Jung, the Swiss pioneer of psycho-analysis, conveyed to me on three occasions through three different mediums that he would like to write through me. Inga was the last of the three and through her he said to me "I need a medium such as you".

As I was already aware of his close connection with us, I felt no hesitation in agreeing to the plan. Having no idea how it was to be done, I had the feeling that it would be great fun. Upon my questioning him, he said that he would not dictate what he wanted to say but "I will give you pure thought which you will formulate into words. The choice of language will be yours. Think about it".

After reflecting for a couple of days and discussing my ideas with Inga, I decided to write in English rather than German and, more precisely, in the type of English which I had used in my practice in the United States with both educated and relatively uneducated people. Any Americanisms not acceptable or comprehensible in Britain could then be edited out by a suitable British typist in consultation with me. The decision about the use of language had an effect similar to setting a computer: The screen, the equivalent of my earth consciousness, received the sentences and paragraphs ready to flow through my pen at great speed without the distraction of any specific awareness of the transmutation process, which was turning the pure, wordless thought into *bona fide* American English.

I did enjoy the process. It started out with a quick jotting down of the chapter headings, followed by Chapter One, and so on. After forty-five to seventy-five minutes the flow would stop, regardless of whether I would have liked to continue. If I tried then to formulate any more ideas with my mind, it felt like trying to start a car which is running out of petrol. What

I produced then was obviously the product of the earthly intellect without assistance from my own higher self or any other, and had to be scratched out because of its dryness and lifelessness.

It did not take me long to figure out that I was being used as a channel under very strict higher-dimensional scientific supervision. The "machine's" energy level and , no doubt, other conditions of which I was unaware were closely monitored. A day or two might pass before I felt the urge to sit down with pen and paper again, or it might happen already on the following day. Meanwhile daily life and work continued. The patients or clients who came were evidently selected by Jung who would then use some of their story as examples in the manuscript as well as drawing on my past clinical experiences.

Between the speed and clarity of his thoughts and my long-established habit of concise verbal expression, the finished manuscript was only booklet-sized. We simply had it reproduced by a local printer, a few hundred at a time. When I read it now I can see how well it stated our collective experience and knowledge of that time, and how much we and the work have evolved since then. May it ever progress and change! Mankind on this planet has suffered long enough from assorted ossifications and fossilisations. Scientific dogma is on exception.

The spirit is flexible and progressive, continuously evolving. It needs to be creative on all levels all the time, free to let go of what is old and outlived, free to receive and handle the new without prejudice.

The older I become, the more I am impressed by the simplicity of man, of truth, of the Universe.

FREE DETAILED CATALOGUE

A detailed illustrated catalogue is available on request, SAE or International Postal Coupon appreciated. **Titles can be ordered direct from Capall Bann, post free in the UK** (cheque or PO with order) or from good bookshops and specialist outlets. Titles currently available include:

Auguries and Omens - The Magical Lore of Birds by Yvonne Aburrow
Caer Sidhe - Celtic Astrology and Astronomy by Michael Bayley
Call of the Horned Piper by Nigel Jackson
Celtic Lore & Druidic Ritual by Rhiannon Ryall
Earth Dance - A Year of Pagan Rituals by Jan Brodie
Earth Magic by Margaret McArthur
Enchanted Forest - The Magical Lore of Trees by Yvonne Aburrow
Familiars - Animal Powers of Britain by Anna Franklin
Healing Book (The) by Chris Thomas
Handbook For Pagan Healers by Liz Joan
Healing Homes by Jennifer Dent
Herbcraft - Shamanic & Ritual Use of Herbs by S Lavender & A Franklin
In Search of Herne the Hunter by Eric Fitch
Magical Lore of Cats by Marion Davies
Magical Lore of Herbs by Marion Davies
Patchwork of Magic by Julia Day
Psychic Self Defence - Real Solutions by Jan Brodie
Sacred Animals by Gordon MacLellan
Sacred Grove - The Mysteries of the Forest by Yvonne Aburrow
Sacred Geometry by Nigel Pennick
Sacred Lore of Horses The by Marion Davies
Secret Places of the Goddess by Philip Heselton
Talking to the Earth by Gordon Maclellan
Taming the Wolf - Full Moon Meditations by Steve Hounsome
VORTEX - The End of History, by Mary Russell

Capall Bann is owned and run by people actively involved in many of the areas in which we publish. Our list is expanding rapidly so do contact us for details on the latest releases.

Capall Bann Publishing, Freshfields, Chieveley, Berks, RG20 8TF